T0146608

The Curious Case of the Alexian Brothers
Behavioral Health Hospital

The Curious Case of the Alexian Brothers Behavioral Health Hospital

And Other Controversies in Psychiatry

Anthony M D'Agostino, MD

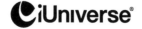

THE CURIOUS CASE OF THE ALEXIAN BROTHERS BEHAVIORAL HEALTH HOSPITAL AND OTHER CONTROVERSIES IN PSYCHIATRY

iUniverse books may be ordered through booksellers or by contacting:

iUniverse
1663 Liberty Drive
Bloomington, IN 47403
www.iuniverse.com
1-800-Authors (1-800-288-4677)

ISBN: 978-1-5320-3780-1 (sc)
ISBN: 978-1-5320-3781-8 (e)

Library of Congress Control Number: 2018906049

Print information available on the last page.

iUniverse rev. date: 08/05/2019

Dedication to

Beverly, Mike, Chris, Jon, Ingrid,
Nico, Celia, and Joseph

CONTENTS

Foreword.. ix

Chapter 1 The Hospital.. 1
Chapter 2 Cellebroeders... 7
Chapter 3 Early Hospitals and Medical Schools 16
Chapter 4 Critical Developments in Surgery,
           Medicine, and Public Health 32
Chapter 5 The Psychiatric Hospital... 44
Chapter 6 Twentieth-Century Medical Interventions in
           Psychiatry before Drugs.. 50
Chapter 7 A Brief History of the Evolution of Health Insurance 70
Chapter 8 Psychiatry Becomes Local.. 76
Chapter 9 Health Insurance, Moral Hazard, and the Market................. 81
Chapter 10 The Ascendancy of Psychoanalysis in American Psychiatry ... 88
Chapter 11 Psychiatry, Health Insurance,
           and the Concept of Moral Hazard 123
Chapter 12 Alexian Brothers Medical Center, 1972–1999.................... 133
Chapter 13 Managed Care Triumphant, or
           "It Depends on What the Meaning of 'Is' Is" 151
Chapter 14 The Trouble with Psychiatry 177

Epilogue 225
References.. 229

FOREWORD

H ow does one weave a literary tapestry that combines historical milestones in psychiatry, the evolution of a compassionate group of Catholic Brothers, political insights to the provision of behavioral health services in an era of turmoil and the emergence of Alexian Brothers Behavioral Health Hospital (ABBHH) as a major force in psychiatric care in 2016. Dr. Anthony D'Agostino has artfully accomplished this task, both from his perspective as a witness to some of these events and a well-read psychiatrist with knowledge about the remainder.

Dr. D'Agostino's credentials are relevant for this task. He served for over 32 years as the Medical Director of Psychiatry at both Alexian Brothers Medical Center and then ABBHH. During this same time he served as President of the Illinois Psychiatric Society, Area representative to the APA and sat on the APA's Managed Care Committee. This relatively brief interval is when a modest psychiatric program in a Catholic sponsored community hospital evolved to become one of the most successful providers of behavioral healthcare in America.

There is a lot of information in this monograph and I was curious how he could touch on so many historical events while keeping the reader's attention. His writing technique seemed erratic at first glance as different time lines were interrupted. However, I am convinced that this technique is what is engaging about his work. There is enough information in this paper to keep a game of Trivial Pursuit going for hours; yet the relations of the Alexian Brothers community in Europe during the Napoleon era is as interesting to read as is the description of general hospital based psychiatric unit closings in the era of managed care and for profit psychiatric facilities. The author's colorful commentary on events also adds to the appeal of his work.

This informative history engages the reader in a refreshing manner that would prove too dry for the average author tackling this project. Dr. D'Agostino not only takes us back over a 600 year time line but also focuses on one of the most eventful and exciting period of this history: the past forty years.

During the critical period of the 1970's through the present, psychiatry evolved from the intellectual grasp of psychoanalysis to embrace DSM III, psychopharmacology, crisis management with cognitive/behavioral therapies and a phasing out of many long stay inpatient services. "Managed Care" not only altered the relationship of patient and doctor but over time has led to radical shifts in how "providers" have to think about market forces and career development. These changes have impacted the psyche of American psychiatrists. Why did this happen and how did ABBHH emerge as a successful organization when others faltered or no longer exist.

During this period Dr. D'Agostino provided the medical leadership of a dynamic team of innovative thinkers committed to success, led by Mark Frey, who understood where behavioral healthcare was heading and how to execute rapid and creative growth strategies during this transition period. While community psychiatric clinics and inpatient units in non-for-profit hospitals shrunk or failed to survive, ABBHH progressively grew to a regional and ultimately national leader in providing behavioral healthcare. There was a reason for this bold expansion and it was rooted in the vision and commitment of the Alexian Brothers themselves.

The Brothers traditionally focused their energy on the sectors of society most neglected and disenfranchised. In the past twenty-five years they embraced the community of adults suffering from AIDS. However, prior to the appearance of AIDS there existed a commitment to the mentally ill that was apparent for centuries in facilities in Europe and later America that utilized a community treatment model that was revolutionary for its time.

It has never been politically popular (and seldom profitable) to care for those who suffer from serious, debilitating and not uncommonly fatal mental illness and chemical dependency. Community hospitals would often have small programs, operating at a loss, to support their local service area. During the past 25 years many of these programs closed as Dr. D'Agostino notes. He provides the reader with a detailed description of why ABBHH was able to achieve a successful outcome in this hostile climate and its continued growth and leadership. As is true of many organizations, it is a combination of the right people, values, commitment and execution.

We are left with a dynamic story woven over 700 years and including a cast of intriguing characters. Dr. D'Agostino has shared his knowledge and experience to allow us insight into the dynamics of the Alexian commitment to the mentally ill as well as how ABBHH has emerged as a leader in behavioral healthcare today.

Gregory A. Teas, MD
Chief of Psychiatry,
Amita Health Network

CHAPTER 1

THE HOSPITAL

On December 1, 2011, an article appeared in the Los Angeles Times reporting that Cedars-Sinai Medical Center, a 958-bed acute care facility with 350 residents, was closing its inpatient and outpatient psychiatric services, including its psychiatric residency training program. There would be some psychiatric services remaining, but only to those inpatients who are primarily there for medical or surgical treatment. In a press release, which purports to answer a question while saying nothing, a hospital spokesperson reported that this decision was driven by "changes to the delivery and organization of healthcare services nationwide."

This is hospitalspeak for the unfortunate reality that either the hospital was incurring unacceptable financial losses in its psychiatric services operation or the profit generated did not justify the direct and indirect costs. It is very unlikely that Cedars-Sinai was unable to find patients for the service. It is very likely that expenses outpaced revenue and they felt the psychiatry service was not worth continuing.

The article goes on to say, "The planned closure is the latest in a long series of reductions in mental health services across the state. California has roughly 6500 acute inpatient psychiatric beds, down from 8500 in 1996 according to the California Hospital Association. There have also been significant cutbacks in Medi-Cal (public aid) funding for mental health services statewide." Jan Emerson-Shea, spokesman for the California Hospital Association, is quoted as saying, "What hospitals across California are grappling with are serious financial challenges that are unrelenting ...

causing hospitals across the state to look at what services they can continue to provide and what services they can't."

Randall Hagar of the California Psychiatric Association is quoted in the same article, saying, "Patients who need psychiatric services are stacking up at the door and have a hard time getting in. It's getting tough out there" (Gorman 2011).

In Illinois, realities are no different. The trend that began about twenty-five years ago has been continuing downward, with poor reimbursement and declining support at all levels. The result has been the downsizing or outright elimination of many freestanding psychiatric hospitals and psychiatric units in general hospitals. Dr. Alex Spadoni, longtime consultant for the Illinois Department of Public Health, has surveyed hospitals in Illinois, comparing bed capacity between 1990 and 2011. In his 2012 report to the Illinois Hospital Association, he calculated that about two thousand beds were lost in Illinois between 1990 and 2011. His reasons include managed care controls, including low per diems and low physician reimbursement; continued reductions (or lack of increases) in Medicare and Medicaid reimbursement; increasing numbers of the uninsured; mental health code complexities; and increasing numbers of psychiatrists abandoning hospital practice.

His list of freestanding (psychiatric) hospital and general hospital psychiatric unit closures include, starting in Chicago, Charter Barclay (123 beds), University (110 beds), St. Elizabeth (70 beds), Sheridan Road (56 beds), Ravenswood (55 beds), Bethany (29 beds), University of Chicago (40 beds before reducing to 22 and then subsequently closing), Lincoln West (26 beds), and Chicago Osteopathic (20 beds).

In the suburbs, trends mirror the city. The list of closed hospitals include Charter, Rockford (60 beds), Rock Creek Center, Lemont (165 beds), Forest Hospital, Des Plaines (142 beds, though some of these had reopened as the Chicago Behavioral Hospital) Old Orchard, Skokie (originally 100 beds, taken over by Presbyterian-St. Luke's and called Rush North Shore at 50 beds and eventually closed), Olympia Fields Hospital Psychiatric service (28 beds), Elmhurst Hospital (20 beds), Loyola (35 beds), St. Francis, Evanston (20 beds), Victory Memorial, Waukegan (52 beds), Condell, Libertyville (20 beds), and Good Shepherd, Barrington (18 beds).

These psychiatric facilities have closed permanently. Others have retained their psychiatric services but with major downsizing. This list includes Lutheran General, Park Ridge (100 to 52 beds), Highland Park (30 to 16 beds), Mercy, Aurora (116 to 56 beds), and so on, including hospitals in downstate Illinois. According to Dr. Spadoni, these two thousand lost beds do not include the many state hospital closures and downsizings, as seen at Chicago Read, Elgin, Tinley Park, and others downstate (Spadoni 2012).

Many general hospitals see psychiatric services as money-losing operations, which are kept open only since options for psychiatric patients at existing facilities elsewhere are diminishing or nonexistent. Some hospitals keep small psychiatric units only so they can hire psychiatrists who are in-house to do psychiatric consultations on medical/surgical patients, which, as with Cedars-Sinai, they deem necessary to appropriately support their medical/surgical populations. Emergency rooms at general hospitals have become default holding facilities for psychiatric patients who have nowhere else to go. State hospitals (at least in Illinois) complain that they're at capacity (and therefore can't take new admissions) while they continue to reduce capacity despite increasing demand and that they cannot (or will not) be resources for the mentally ill filling the emergency rooms of local general hospitals.

Modern Healthcare, on November 18, 2013, highlighted the problem of decreasing psychiatric bed capacity. In an article titled "Bedding, Not Boarding," it detailed the phenomenon of psychiatric patients boarding in hospital emergency rooms, sometimes for weeks at a time, waiting for psychiatric beds to open somewhere. According to this article, a congressional staff briefing in March 2012 by the National Association of State Mental Health Program Directors, reporting on a survey of more than six thousand emergency departments nationwide, found that 70 percent of emergency rooms reported boarding psychiatric patients for hours or days, and 10 percent reported often boarding patients for several weeks. The article goes on to point out that

> nationwide, closures reduced the number of beds available in the combined 50 states to 28 percent of the number considered necessary for minimally adequate inpatient psychiatric services. A minimum of 50 beds per 100,000 populations, nearly three times the current bed population,

is a consensus target for providing minimally adequate treatment. (By way of comparison, the ratio in England in 2008 was 63.2 per 100,000 population).

Between 2009 and 2012, an additional 3,222 state hospital beds were closed, and more are planned, according to the article's author (Kutscher 2013).

State-run psychiatric hospital beds were 43,318 in 2010, or 14 per 100,000 people, compared with 50,509 in 2005 and 560,000 in 1955. The article reported that psychiatric patients waiting in emergency departments cost a hospital about $100 per hour in addition to suffering declines in quality of care, patient satisfaction, and public reputation occasioned by longer waiting times for medical/surgical patients.

More than fifty years ago, there were large state hospitals for those who needed them. Where health insurance does exist, major profits now go mostly to large insurance companies, whereas in the past they went to a hospital, which explains the dwindling availability of private sector beds. Government-funded programs like Medicare are basically break-even enterprises or, in the case of public aid, money-losing activities for most hospitals, with the exception of those hospitals operated almost exclusively for those on public aid. Under the Affordable Care Act, often referred to derisively as Obamacare, these too may gradually (or maybe not so gradually) fade away.

All of this makes the Alexian Brothers Behavioral Health Hospital in Hoffman Estates, Illinois, something of a curiosity at this time in history. Purchased in February 1999 from for-profit Hospital Corporation of America (HCA), it had 95 beds and a census of perhaps 7 to 10 patients (reports vary) in the entire facility on the February 1999 closing date. HCA was, reportedly, losing roughly $200,000 to $250,000 per month in the previous year.

Alexian Brothers Medical Center, located nine miles southeast of the newly purchased psychiatric hospital, had a psychiatric division with 55 beds before closing and moving to the new facility. A few years later, bed capacity was increased from 95 to 137 and later to 141.

Eleven years later, the March 2010 issue of Modern Healthcare listed the Alexian Brothers Behavioral Health Hospital as the eleventh-largest psychiatric health care organization in the United States. Ahead of it on the list were two for-profit hospital corporations: Psychiatric Solutions, operating 73 hospitals with 6,423 beds, and Universal Health Services, with 51 hospitals and 4,656 beds. The others comprised a number of other quite large, usually multihospital organizations or large health plans, such as Boston's Partners HealthCare or the Sheppard Pratt Health System outside of Baltimore, which has been in the psychiatric care business for more than 125 years, operating two hospitals with 522 beds and associated outpatient facilities as of the end of 2009.

In 2010, Universal Health Services bought out Psychiatric Solutions, creating a single organization operating 9,937 beds as the largest psychiatric corporate entity in the country. That merger brought Alexian Brothers to tenth place in the nation by the end of 2010.

As of the February 2012 issue of Modern Healthcare, Alexian Brothers was now ranked seventh in the nation. What makes this noteworthy is that, at the time of the 2010 publication, Alexian Brothers was operating out of a single location in Hoffman Estates, Illinois, located thirty-five miles northwest of downtown Chicago, with 137 beds and an outpatient office next door. In 2010, bed capacity was increased to 141, and two rather small outpatient satellites were added. How what was in 1999 a 55-bed psychiatric facility housed in a condemned former nursing home (the state of Illinois felt the building was too dilapidated and no longer met code for patient habitation) at a 400-bed community hospital in 1998 got to number seven in the nation might be a story worth examining in its own right, as well as a reflection of changing trends in mental health care and funding over the last three decades.

In 2013, the Alexian Brothers Behavioral Health Hospital admitted 6,355 inpatients (turning away over 800 for lack of capacity), registered 3,863 day-hospital patients (37,559 visits), and counted 2,133 intensive outpatient admissions (19,789 visits). The hospital performed 2,837 ECT treatments (many referred from outside the system from hospitals lacking capacity and facilities), in addition to 84,899 individual and family outpatient office visits at its two outpatient office locations in Hoffman Estates and Elk Grove Village. The intake department, known as Access, did 16,764 individual patient evaluations to assess the appropriate level of care to which patients were referred.

Its clinical research division participated in numerous clinical drug

5

trials and implanted twenty patients (over a four-year period) as part of a clinical trial of deep brain stimulation for patients suffering from intractable depression. It is the largest private psychiatric organization in Illinois (according to Modern Healthcare) in terms of patient activity, although in terms of bed capacity, it is not the largest in Illinois.

Modern Healthcare based its rankings on what it refers to as "net patient revenue." As a freestanding hospital, it cannot receive payment for any adult on public aid. However, about 35 percent of its child/adolescent admissions are paid for by public aid, and approximately 10 percent of all admissions to the facility are patients with no health insurance of any kind, subsidized by the Alexian Brothers Health System.

In an attempt to understand the how and why of this kind of growth in psychiatric services since 1999, in what appears to be a climate of dwindling support, one needs to examine both internal and external factors. An important factor has been changes in the way psychiatric and other medical services have been paid for over the past thirty years. In any transitional period, in any kind of enterprise, how the organization manages or otherwise responds to those changes determines who survives (or chooses to survive) and who does not. In the not-for-profit world of health care, "mission" as well as "community need" are supposed to play central roles, and they generally do. But, as one sees with Cedars-Sinai Medical Center and the multitude of closed and downsized hospitals in Illinois, no organization is going to lose money indefinitely, nor should they be expected to do so.

To begin this story, it may be of interest to review some of the historical antecedents from which hospitals in general, and this Alexian Brothers Hospital in particular, have evolved. In the fast-paced, high-stakes business that health care has become, there may be value in looking at where we've been, how we got there, where we want to go, and why we want to go there.

CHAPTER 2

CELLEBROEDERS

The story of this Alexian Brothers facility has to begin with the Alexian Brothers themselves, a Catholic religious order that began some seven (probably eight) hundred years ago, apparently as a lay religious movement centering in the cities of Aachen and Cologne in what is now Germany, and Antwerp in what is now Belgium. Whether these groups prior to about 1320 were in communication with each other or just shared similar missions is unclear. Alexian historian Lawrence Davidson (1990) reports that by 1859, the Alexian congregation had been in Aachen for 529 years. The focus appears to have been in the cities, since that's where the needs were most acute, according to Davidson, as the urban proletariat began to evolve.

Ministering to the sick poor was a primary mission of these laymen, who chose to own no property and to live a communal life devoted to service to the community. It was their belief that Christ had instructed his apostles to live in this way, but that the established church had strayed substantially from that original directive. This way of life was based on the account of St. Luke (himself a physician) of the early church in Jerusalem. In his gospel and in the Acts of the Apostles, according to Alexian historian Christopher Kauffman (1976), "Luke stressed Jesus's love of sinners, his forgiveness, and his loving concern for the impoverished lower classes in contrast to his severe attitude toward those self-righteous aristocrats who abused their power and wealth." These ideas were considered revolutionary in Roman times, as well as in the fourteenth century.

According to Kauffman, "we know of no one founder, no early rule, no chapter meetings, and they left us neither letters nor diaries." The absence of written records before about 1350 suggests most likely a lack of skill in reading and writing among the "poor men" (men of the lower classes), as they were known, who participated in this essentially lay movement.

These early Alexians were considered suspect by the established church since they were thought to be "associated with a reform reaction against the abuses of the church, particularly the secularism of the clergy … Because they were also harassed by local bishops and papal inquisitors, the charge of heresy played a major role in their early history" (Kauffman). There is reference, going back to 1259, of a decree implying that they might be potential heretics. There is another reference to 1307 referred to by Kauffmann excommunicating the brothers of the Lungengasse in Cologne, although the ban was lifted in 1308 when some influential citizens of the city came to their defense. It wasn't until 1472 that the Brothers, called Cellites during this period (a reference to the architecture of their houses, which contained "cells" where individual Brothers slept), became an order formally sanctioned by the papacy. The "Alexian" name came later.

Up to 1472, the Brothers in each city were considered under the authority of their local parishes. As a formally sanctioned order they could now be independent of local parishes and build their own chapels, after tactful negotiations with local bishops. The first was consecrated in Aachen on January 1, 1477. It was dedicated to Saints Augustine and Alexius. The new order's rule (analogous to an organization's bylaws) was adopted from the Augustinians, who acted as consultants of sorts now that the organization was "official." On May 6, 1491, the Brothers in Antwerp were granted permission to build their own chapel independent of the local parish. In 1493, it was completed and took St. Alexius as its patron saint. In Cologne, a chapel wasn't constructed until 1508; it was consecrated to St. Alexius on the second Sunday after Easter. Since the Brothers in each city had adopted St. Alexius as their common patron, they eventually became known as Alexian Brothers.[1]

---

[1] The Alexian Brothers' entry into health care came not as a curative mission so much as a palliative one, a "death with dignity" ministry, which continues to this day in the United States in the form of the Alexian Brothers Aids Ministry. The original purpose of this ministry was essentially the same as it was in 1347 (i.e., to establish humane, residential programs in the Chicago area for patients who had

Even before the arrival of the Black Death (bubonic plague) in Northern Europe in 1347, digging graves and burying the dead were apparently a couple of their duties, along with caring for the sick and the infirm, primarily in their own homes. Grave digging was not a profession high on the social hierarchy of the times, and their primary source of income came from begging.

After the arrival of the Black Death, coming initially between 1347 and 1350, the population of Europe was devastated with an estimated twenty million deaths. The needs were so acute and the resources so scarce that city councils in some areas funded the efforts of these groups who cared for the sick and buried the dead. The Alexian Brothers' logo contains two crossed shovels meant to call attention to the fact that one of their missions was to bury the legions of dead left as sequelae of the Black Death.

While the modes of transmission in infectious disease weren't fully understood for another five hundred years, even the unlettered poor of Europe understood that contact with victims of plague had something to do with the spread of disease. As a result, victims were cared for and/or buried, to the extent possible, outside city walls (hence the term "outsiders") and shunned by the populace at large and even by relatives. It took uncommon faith and a willingness to adhere to the "mission" to voluntarily expose oneself to plague in order to provide a proper Christian burial. It was hard physical labor but did not require years of education; the work was seen as an "Imitation of Christ" by its practitioners.

As the centuries progressed, the Alexian Brothers' ministry became more clearly focused on providing care for the sick poor, whether the sickness was engendered by plagues, old age, or other naturally occurring maladies, such as mental illnesses. Most care of the sick occurred in the home, but some patients, especially the mentally ill, often required institutional care.

The earliest document associating the Alexian Brothers with institutional care for the mentally ill is from 1569 in the city of Nijmegen (Holland) where one Petre de Hoogh was directed by the city council to stay with the "Cellebroeders," as they were still known at the time. In

---

AIDS [plague] and were expected to die). With the advent of the new antiviral drugs for HIV-positive patients, fewer people actually die of AIDS these days. Nevertheless, the Alexian-supported residential programs for HIV-positive patients have expanded in recent years, of which there are currently three in the Chicago area.

1585, according to Kauffman (1978), there's reference to a woman "oiver viff sinnen beroefft" (bereft of her senses) who was confined to the Cellite house. By 1592, the Brothers in Nijmegen became known for their care of "kranckzinnighe menschen" (mentally ill men). From that year the Brothers' house in that city was called a "dolhuys" (madhouse). There was another dolhuys in Braunschweig operated by the Brothers.

Many considered mental illness during this period as a moral (residuals continue today in the form of stigma) rather than a medical issue and often understood as a consequence of "turning away" from God. The sometimes-unrestrained expression of sexual and aggressive impulses at times probably seemed to lend support to that view. A source of income in sixteenth-century mental institutions (more famously at "Bedlam" in London and elsewhere) was the charging of admission to allow local townsfolk to view the insane, sometimes housed in cages. Parents would bring their children so they could view firsthand the ravages of immorality. Apparently the Alexian house in Nijmegen at first was no exception and had visitors early on, though in the Alexian archives there is a reference to this practice being soon discontinued (Kauffman 1978). Unruly crowds, especially children, became an impediment to what the Brothers felt was proper care for this population. However, in the fifteenth and sixteenth centuries, there is no record of the houses in Aachen, Antwerp, or Cologne dealing with any significant numbers of mentally ill until the time of the French Revolution, although that ministry was apparently well established by 1789. There is evidence that the Alexian houses in those three cities (in centuries before the French Revolution) functioned as small hospices for wayward boys, and priests in need of what Kauffmann refers to as "moral reform," along with a few mental patients.[2]

The Enlightenment of the eighteenth century began to change the public's conception of the mentally ill to that of victims of illness, although that view evolved rather slowly despite the revolutionary zeal of reformers.

---

[2] In the 1790s France the confiscation of the lands of the Nobility and the Clergy formed the basis of French paper money, the Assignat. Inflation is a great help in financing war, and the idea was to sell the land to redeem the paper money. Printing more money than land sales could support was irresistible in the short term and results in inflation, which is bad for the population at large but good for those who owe money (like the government).

Napoleon's plan apparently was to spread quasi-Enlightenment ideas (while taking the title of emperor) by conquering most of Europe and making some of it part of France. By 1802, Aachen, Cologne, and Antwerp were indeed parts of France. However, the anticlerical and militantly secular (radicals wanted to de-Christianize France) mood of the French Revolution resulted in the confiscation of the Alexian properties between 1794 and 1802, primarily to help finance Napoleon's many wars. The Alexian houses in the Netherlands and the Rhineland were either closed or used to billet French soldiers. That they were allowed to exist at all was because they were deemed "socially useful." With morale low and their assets mostly gone, it seemed that five hundred years might be as far as the Cellebroeders would go.

After the defeat of Napoleon in 1814, Aachen and Cologne became part of Protestant Prussia, and Antwerp became part of a Dutch state under the Dutch Protestant King William I. What that meant in practical terms was that the defeat of Napoleon did not result in the restoration of Alexian assets. In 1830, the Belgians separated from Holland to create an independent, primarily Catholic, Belgium. Aachen and Cologne remained part of Prussia, which, in the 1870s and later, busied itself in the creation of the modern German state.

Nationalism was one of the many isms of the time (1848 and later), and German Chancellor Otto von Bismarck's goal (1870s) was to focus all German loyalties in the newly Prussianized German state. The Lutheran church was the official state church in the new Germany, and, as was the case in most official state churches, the local king (or kaiser) was head of the church as well as of the state. Catholics posed a problem in that their religious loyalties were not necessarily synonymous with the goals of the nation-state. Moreover, after the Franco-Prussian War (1870–1871), part of what now was Germany was French speaking and formerly part of France (Alsace-Lorraine), and Bismarck was suspicious of their loyalties.

In the movement known as the Kulturkampf, beginning in 1871, a series of laws were passed to weaken the influence of the Catholic church in Germany. According to Kauffman, "the Catholic Department within the Ministry of Public Worship and Education was abolished and all Catholic schools were placed under state supervision. The Jesuit and the Redemptorist Orders were dissolved and forced into exile. The Pulpit Law ... was aimed at preventing Catholics from antistate preaching." In

1875, laws were passed "whereby all houses and institutions maintained by religious orders, except those engaged in nursing the sick, were dissolved." Thousands of religious were forced into exile, and approximately one thousand parishes were without priests. As it turned out, however, it only succeeded in uniting German Catholics and strengthened the Catholic center party, which increased its strength in the Reichstag. Bismarck then decided that a Catholic anti-German conspiracy was, perhaps, not really a major threat, and after 1880 enforcement gradually diminished.

During this period the Alexians evolved into an organization whose mission in Europe became, more and more, the care of the mentally ill. Asylums, it seems, were apolitical. Although traditional nursing functions remained, mostly in the homes of patients, the Brothers' function as buriers of the dead and managers of cemeteries diminished as the secular state took over these functions.

During the nineteenth century, the Alexians adopted what was the dominant school of thought among German psychiatrists, which was that mental illness is a form of disease of the brain. As the nineteenth century progressed, German medicine in general and psychiatry in particular began to supplant the French, who were the undisputed leaders in medicine earlier in the century.

According to Zilboorg (1941),

> the creative genius of the German psychiatrist seems to have risen to the needs of his day with more than creditable efficiency and dispatch. The work of non-restraint (working with unchained patients) alone-a matter of struggle, contention, and bureaucratic obstacles in many parts of France and England-was carried out in the greater part of Germany almost without difficulty … The German hospital became an institution for treatment and research … almost within one generation. Nowhere in the world during the middle part of the century was so much research done in Psychiatry as in Germany.

Mental health care expanded rapidly in Germany in the late nineteenth century. Zilboorg reports that in Prussia in 1852 there were nineteen private asylums, in 1872 there were forty-eight, and in 1886 the number was eighty-six. According to Burdett (1891), "the largest (asylum) is that of the Alexianer Brethren in Aix-la-Chapelle (Aachen), with 310 beds." It remains in existence today.

By the end of the nineteenth century, the Brothers had asylums or general hospitals in Aachen; Henri-Chapelle; Krefeld; München-Gladbach; Munster; Cologne; Chicago; St. Louis; Oshkosh, Wisconsin; Elizabeth, New Jersey; as well as facilities in England, Switzerland, Ireland, and Northern Ireland.

According to the Constitution of the Alexian Brothers (West Chester, NY, 1878), the following are the rules for the "care of the insane":

1. Every Brother should look upon the insane who are entrusted to his care, as beings whose unusually helpless condition claims a greater share of Christian charity, and for whose security and welfare he must labor to the best of his power, for the love of God, whose image they still retain in their souls.

2. In order that a Brother may fulfill his duties toward the insane … he should know how to govern himself … he should never suffer himself to be carried away by impatience, anger, fear or other disorderly movements of the soul … but always preserve a uniform tranquility of mind … That he may do this more easily, let him reflect that whatever, in the conduct of these unfortunate beings, might provoke him to anger, should be looked upon as merely a manifestation of their disease; and hence that even if they burst out into violent bursts of passion, or into furious complaints and calumnies, nay, even should they attack him … he should look upon all this as the conduct of men who are not responsible for it.

3. Every Brother should make it a constant rule to treat the insane with kindness and love … It is never allowed to lay violent hands on an insane person … Brothers are allowed to defend themselves, provided they observe due moderation in their defense, from the attacks of furious madman; but in this case they must intend nothing more than to deprive such persons, and that with all gentleness, of the power of doing injury.

4. Every insane person should be treated with that care and civility which are due to his estate and condition, just as though he were of sound mind. Abusive expressions … should never be heard from the lips of a Brother.

5. When the insane persons give vent to foolish or delirious language, or when they are disturbed by strange phantoms of the imagination endeavor to quiet them with kind words … if he sees that he cannot pacify them with words of kindness, he should be silent.

6. The Brothers should keep a watchful eye upon their patients day and night, lest the latter hurt themselves or others, or injure or destroy their clothing, bedding, food, etc.

7. With regard to food, linen, occupation, recreation and medicines, the Brothers should comply strictly with the physician, and, at every visit, they should give him an accurate account of whatever they have observed in the patients.

8. When food is put into the cell of those who are furiously mad and violent, the Brother should see that they eat, and observe the quantity that they eat. He should attend with particular care to such as refuse all nourishment for a considerable time, especially when they manifest an intention to starve themselves … he should refer the matter to the Rector, who shall obtain the personal aid of the physician.

9. They should get possession of no utensils or instruments with which they might harm themselves or others; or at least such things must be given only with great discretion …

10. The taking of medicines should never be left entirely to the patient, but the Brother should watch that the remedies be taken, or administer them with his own hand.

11. When a Brother notices that any of the patients under his charge has disappeared, he should inform the Rector, whose duty it is to see that the necessary measures be taken.

12. It is the duty of the Rector to provide that insane persons be never left to themselves, but that a Brother be always with them and watch over them.

13. The strictest care should be had over such insane persons as are led by blind instinct to the commission of indecent actions. They should be prevented, as much as possible, from doing such things, and especially from drawing others to do the same by their example.

From mental illness as a moral problem to mental illness as a medical problem, what a difference a few hundred years can make!

CHAPTER 3

EARLY HOSPITALS AND MEDICAL SCHOOLS

Many religious orders in the past served the functions of what today we would refer to as social service agencies. Care for the sick and the poor has always been a community need and was financed by the age-old practice of begging or by some more formal contract with local city authorities. Through the agency of the church, it has always been considered the obligation of the wealthy to support the sick and the poor. Hospitals evolved out of early almshouses basically as places where the sick poor sometimes came to get treatment, such as it was, but more often simply to die or to be cared for when they couldn't care for themselves. Up to almost the turn of the twentieth century, few people, especially if they had means, went to a hospital. Physicians came to them. The bulk of sick patients were treated in the home and either recovered or died there, but few chose a hospital if they could avoid it. Hospitals were where the poor folks went.

Most of the care of the sick by Alexian Brothers prior to 1850 was home care, although institutional psychiatric care had been well established by that time. Except in very rare cases, hospitals were not institutions highly regarded by the public. Recall that when President Abraham Lincoln was shot in April 1865, and despite all that was learned about gunshot wounds in the Civil War, no one seemed to have thought to take him to a hospital. Of the hundreds of cowboy films and thousands of shoot-outs personally witnessed on the silver screen as a child growing up in the 1940s and early 1950s, I never saw any cowboy (or Indian, for that matter) taken to a hospital.

The Alexian Brothers in Europe today operate about 4,500 psychiatric, physical rehab (called neurology hospitals), and general medical beds in Germany, in addition to hospitals in other countries. The psychiatric ministry encompasses all levels of care from acute to rehabilitative to custodial care of the chronic and persistently mentally ill. During a 2008 visit to the Alexian facilities in Germany, a group from the Alexian Brothers Behavioral Health Hospital in Hoffman Estates, Illinois, visited a cemetery on the grounds of a psychiatric hospital in Munster, where the Brothers, and the patients they cared for, were buried together in the same cemetery.

In the former East Berlin, we visited an Alexian general medical hospital as well as an Alexian psychiatric facility that apparently were in operation throughout the communist era, as well as many years before, and now since. The need goes on despite whatever political ideology is in vogue at the time. It doesn't take great insight to see that this is a long-term ministry and not a short-term exploitation of a "market."

The Alexian Brothers in the United States eventually became an independent organization, having now only a traditional/sentimental relationship to their German origins. Initially, however, they were very closely tied to Aachen (Germany at the time did not yet exist as a specific country). When Brother Bonaventure Thelen was sent here in 1866, the American Civil War concluded, and opened their first US facility in Chicago, it was meant to serve the needs of a primarily German-speaking population. These early hospitals were general medical facilities, but with room made for psychiatric patients, as was their practice in Europe. Here the Brothers cared for the gamut of medical and psychiatric needs of primarily male patients.

In most of the larger nineteenth-century hospitals, patients were cared for in "wards," a term only recently abandoned in American hospitals. The single-bed room had not yet arrived, and curtains, if they had any privacy at all, might separate patients, as was the case in the mega-hospitals found most notably in Paris, London, and Vienna before 1860. Large wards are still found in many countries around the world, even relatively advanced countries like Great Britain.

There were usually separate male and female wards in most hospitals. The large ward with forty or fifty (primarily male) patients in a single very large room I have only encountered personally at Cook County Hospital in Chicago as a medical student in the early sixties and, to a lesser extent, at the Los Angeles County General Hospital, as an intern in 1965–1966. Female wards at Cook County Hospital were usually smaller, but twelve-bed wards were common. Controlling infection among patients in these open conditions must have been challenging and perhaps contributed to the public's fear of hospitals.

In those wards everyone was exposed to everyone. Modesty and privacy usually took a back seat to necessity. Since nursing personnel at the early Alexian hospitals were all Brothers, taking care of females was apparently deemed inappropriate. These early hospitals were basically monasteries (or convents in the case of nuns) attached to a health care facility. For this reason the Alexian Brothers hospitals in Chicago, and later in St. Louis, were for men only and remained so in Chicago until as late as 1962. In more modern times this practice had a limiting effect on growth and forced the hospital's medical staff to hospitalize female patients elsewhere. Obviously, obstetrics and gynecology were not available services at early Alexian Brothers hospitals.

There was very little profit to be gained operating hospitals in the nineteenth century and before, which is how the various religious organizations (and local/national governments) came to be in the hospital business in the first place. Not-for-profit then was a literal truth before it became a legal definition. Nevertheless, after about 1850, the concept of the hospital as a place to actually treat the sick, as opposed to simply isolating them to protect the healthy, began to take hold in America, though very slowly. In most of Europe it was rather different, especially in major capitals like Paris, Vienna, London, and Berlin.

In the medical world of the first half of the nineteenth century, Paris was in a class all its own. The hospital system developed by the French after the 1789 Revolution (but begun even earlier) was unmatched anywhere and set the standard for the world. It would take another sixty years or more before coming to most countries, including the United States. Historian David McCullough's book The Greater Journey: Americans in Paris (2011), devotes chapter 4 to describing the hospitals of Paris in the 1830s:

> The largest was the HOTEL DIEU (originally founded in 1602) at 1,400 beds, consisted of two buildings on

opposite banks of the Seine. They were five-stories high and were connected by a covered bridge. It was considered pre-eminent in surgery. It treated 15,000 patients a year. A short distance away the HOPITAL de la PITIE, at 800 beds, specialized in clinical medicine especially diseases of the chest, which in those times meant primarily tuberculosis.

At about 400 beds stood the HOPITAL de la CHARITE and also the first children's hospital in the world, HOPITAL des INFANTES MALADIES. Mental disorders had their own hospitals, the SALPETRIERE for women (where Freud studied "hysteria" under the French Neurologist Charcot) and the BICETRE for men. There was even a hospital specializing in diseases of the skin; again, the first in the world.

McCullough reports that in 1833, the twelve hospitals of Paris treated 65,935 patients. By contrast, the best medical and psychiatric hospitals in America, Massachusetts General and McLain, both in Boston, treated fewer than 800 between them.

In terms of medical education, America had nothing to compare to Paris's Ecole de Medecine (school of medicine) founded in 1776. In 1830s America there were only twenty-one medical schools, with faculties of only five or six professors, if they were lucky. The twenty-one schools together enrolled about 2,500 students, with the vast majority of physicians in the United States never attending medical school at all. Shorter (1997) quotes historian Rosemary Stevens: "In 1900 less than 10 percent of practicing physicians in the USA were graduates of genuine medical schools. About 20 percent had never attended medical school lectures. The majority were the products of apprenticeships or of the proprietary schools." Little wonder why studying in Europe was so highly valued.

The Ecole de Medecine in Paris enrolled 5,000 students with a full-time (paid by the government) faculty of twenty-six who lectured on "Anatomy, Physiology, Physics, Medical Hygiene, Medical Natural History, Accouchements (birth), Surgical Pathology, Pharmacology and Organic

Chemistry, Medical Pathology, Therapeutics, Pathological Anatomy, Operative Surgery, Clinical Surgery, Clinical Medicine, Clinical Midwifery, Diseases of Women and Children, and Legal Medicine." Classes were in French (as opposed to Latin) to allow the children of tradesmen and peasants to attend if they could make the grade, and many did. Admission to this medical school required a college degree or equivalent (an extraordinary standard at the time), but foreigners (like Americans) were exempt from this requirement. All courses and lectures were free of charge, another French revolutionary innovation to encourage higher education among the commoners.

In America there was nothing to compare to the teaching and plethora of clinical material all within a few blocks or miles of each other, which is why American students went to Paris to study medicine if they could at all afford it. Oliver Wendell Holmes, better known as a writer and poet and one of the founders of the literary magazine Atlantic Monthly, was first a physician and wrote many letters home chronicling his experiences. He stayed about two years and finally came home when ordered by his father to do so. Study in Paris brought great prestige among a physician's peers in America at the time.

Nursing in Paris was also in a class all its own. Nurses were mostly all nuns of the Order of St. Augustine, the Soers de la Charité (Daughters of Charity) who wore large white caps that were later to evolve into nurse's caps, which became symbolic of the profession (when it became a profession). In the United States these caps were later individualized according to the hospital or school where the nurse trained. Although the postrevolutionary French governments were anticlerical, nursing in those days was full-time all the time and required twenty-four-hour dedication. The American students were greatly impressed by their skill and dedication, according to McCullough (2011). The hospital-oriented nursing profession was developed here, and when in England a professional nursing core was developed, nurses there were also called "sisters" (the term "nurse" in a medical context was to come later) after the French model even though they were not Catholic nuns.

Although by this time in history surgery was becoming a respected and prestigious profession, there was still no general anesthesia as we know it, and no sterile technique, even in enlightened Paris. McCullough tells of

Mason Warren, a Paris medical student and son of Massachusetts General Hospital surgeon John Collins Warren, who wrote his father that about two-thirds of all patients operated on, even by the most skilled surgeons, died, usually of infection. Warren wrote to his father of one case done by the illustrious surgeon Philibert Roux, who insisted on removing a tumor from an elderly man who died an hour later. Warren estimated that the man would have lived five or six years longer without the surgery. Since patients paid no fees for their care, Dr. Roux's motive for doing the surgery was that doing difficult surgeries challenged him, and the tumor, like Mount Everest, was simply there and needed to be attempted, "the surgery was a success but the patient unfortunately died." Alas, one likes to believe that medical science was somehow served by these exploits, even though, inevitably, some harm occurred as surgeons explored various procedures and techniques to treat what seemed to need treating.

Even without surgery, studying medicine was still a very messy affair. Composer Hector Berlioz (1990) was a medical student in Paris in the 1820s and kept a record of his experiences. In his memoirs he left an account of his first visit to the dissecting room at the Hospice de la Pitie:

> At the sight of that terrible charnel-house – the fragments of limbs, the grinning faces and gaping skulls, the bloody quagmire underfoot and the atrocious smell it gave off, the swarms of sparrows wrangling over scraps of lung, the rats in their corner gnawing the bleeding vertebrae-such a feeling of revulsion possessed me that I leapt through the window of the dissecting-room and fled for home as though Death and all his hideous train were at my heels. The shock of that first impression lasted for twenty-four hours. I did not want to hear another word about anatomy, dissection or medicine, I meditated a hundred mad schemes of escape from the future that hung over me.

Like most medical students, he eventually got over the horror but then took a different path.

Meanwhile, back in frontier Chicago in 1850, physicians from Rush Medical College, the first and one of the more progressive medical schools in the city at that time, opened a twelve-bed hospital meant to enhance clinical teaching opportunities (Bonner 1991). It was called the Illinois General Hospital of the Lakes at Rush and Water Streets. The charge was three dollars per week per patient. The doctors asked a Catholic religious order, the Sisters of Mercy (following the French model), to provide nursing care and in 1851 transferred control of the facility to the nuns. The doctors were not necessarily Catholics, but they saw that nuns running hospitals, in a world without health insurance, was a very cost-effective way to operate a medical facility. It was later renamed Mercy Hospital and still exists as Chicago's oldest continuously running hospital currently at Twenty-Sixth and Calumet. Nuns, like with the Brothers, provided a reliable, dedicated, and inexpensive labor supply.

Before moving to Elk Grove Village in 1966, there were four previous Alexian hospitals on Chicago's North Side, which early on was an area of major German settlement. This followed a typical ethnic-religious pattern common in Chicago and elsewhere. Since the early Brothers were from Germany, the population served here, at least at first, was largely German-speaking (Davidson 1990).

Most hospitals in Chicago and other large Midwestern and Eastern cities had some religious affiliation and sponsorship, which closely followed ethnic origins and were built in neighborhoods populated by those ethnic groups (venture capital would not be a factor for another hundred years). In Chicago, Swedish Covenant, Norwegian American (Lutheran), Mount Sinai and Michael Reese (Jewish), the Presbyterian Hospital, and St. Luke's Hospital (Episcopal) were typical of the trends. I came into the world at Mother Cabrini Hospital operated by an order of Italian Catholic nuns on the near West Side. Just down the street from Mother Cabrini was Hull House, where Jane Addams worked to create the new profession of social work.

At what became Northwestern University Medical School, the Wesley Pavilion was originally the Methodist Wesley Memorial Hospital, established in 1888 (Shorter 1997, Bonner 1991). The Passavant Pavilion, originally named the Emergency Hospital, was built in 1884 after the original Deaconess Hospital (Lutheran) burned down in the Chicago Fire of 1871. It acquired the Passavant name in honor of the Lutheran pastor who founded these hospitals, William Passavant. In 1920, Passavant became a clinical site for Northwestern University, and in 1941, Methodist Wesley Hospital joined Passavant as part of Northwestern's medical campus.

With a very large Catholic population, Chicago naturally had (and continues to have) many Catholic hospitals, depending on the original ethnicity of the served populations. The historical association between organized religion and health care obviously goes back many centuries. Hospitals primarily served the poor of their respective communities. The juxtaposition of social need and the ability of organized religion to respond to community need, especially in those times when hospitals were essentially expensive charitable ventures, spoke to the social usefulness of these organizations.

Most, but not all, of Chicago's recent arrivals were from Europe or of European ancestry. In 1891, one of the first African American surgeons in Chicago, Daniel Hale Williams, established Provident Hospital on Chicago's South Side. Its purpose was to ensure hospital services to Chicago's African American population and to provide a place where African American doctors and health care workers might practice and learn since they were often excluded at other hospitals.

The Alexian Brothers' first "hospital" was a small house at Schiller and Dearborn (Davidson 1990). It had only eight beds. It opened in June 1866, just in time for yet another outbreak of cholera in the city. Patients were plentiful from the start such that by 1867 it was apparent that eight beds weren't going to suffice. By this time there were six Brothers in Chicago. They looked around for another property and found it at the corner of Franklin and Market Streets, sold to them by William Butler Ogden, mayor of Chicago in 1837 and first president of the Union Pacific Railroad in 1862.

The price was $10,000, and he donated $1,000, so the Brothers received the property for $9,000 to be paid out over four years at 6 percent interest. The building itself cost an additional $30,000. This second hospital was built in 1868 and had seventy beds but burned to the ground three years later, as did many other hospitals, in the great Chicago Fire of 1871.

The third hospital, completed in 1873, had 170 beds and was further enlarged in 1888. It was during the years between 1860 and 1900 that hospitals everywhere were being rapidly transformed, through the influence medical science, into our more contemporary notions of what hospitals should be.

In the1890s, the Chicago Elevated Railway (the "L") was being built and, as luck would have it, would run right through the Alexian Brothers' third hospital property. After some legal maneuverings and legal threats on both sides, the Brothers sold it to the railroad for around $200,000 and used that money to buy land farther north at Belden and Racine Avenues and built yet another hospital in 1898.

In that year, the School of Nursing was established to train Brothers to do more professional nursing, as nursing began to evolve into a true profession, as opposed to simply a core of hardworking humanitarian volunteers. Since income from patients was at best meager and at worst nonexistent, cows were kept and vegetables grown to make sure everyone ate as regularly as possible. To continue in operation, the position of "Brother Collector" came into being and was practiced with reasonable success, which was how expansion became possible. Hospital fund-raising is almost as important today as it was then as a source of capital for most not-for-profit hospitals.

Debt was a major source of contention between the Alexian Brothers in America and those in Germany since more debt meant more fund-raising. Fund-raising required contact with the worldly (and the secular) and left less time for prayer and work. Debt was a four-letter word in Germany at the time, but in America Brother Bonaventure Thelen understood the need to borrow money if growth was to continue.

For reasons lost in Chicago's sometimes-murky, albeit colorful, history, the Alexian Brothers Hospital at Belden and Racine developed a reputation for working well with the Chicago Police (Davidson 1990). It is not known for sure, but one idea was that the Brothers were not overly fussy about payment and, being a male-only hospital, were likely to accept the rougher elements of Chicago society. For example, in the case of a shooting (not an uncommon occurrence then, as now), the practice was to bring the victim to the Alexian hospital, if only to be pronounced dead before transporting him to the Cook County Morgue.

So it came to pass on that infamous St. Valentine's Day in 1929, when the bodies of seven unfortunate associates of the Irish bootlegger Bugs Moran were found inside the SMC Cartage Company garage on North Clark Street. When the bodies arrived at the Alexian Brothers

Hospital, there was only one man still alive. Brother Vincent Geist was there to witness and record the encounter when the police brought in Frank "Louie" Gusenberg, who police hoped could identify the shooters (who were themselves dressed as police officers; Dahl 2012). According to Brother Vincent, Louie's last words were "Get out of here, and let me die in peace." His request was apparently granted, and he died shortly after arrival.

Once again in 1934, police drove the bullet-ridden body of John Dillinger past three hospitals—Augustana, Grant (formerly known as the German Hospital), and St. Joseph—to the Alexian Brothers Hospital after he was dispatched by the FBI from this life to whatever lay beyond for unrepentant bank robbers (Dahl 2012). These events are mentioned only to highlight the obvious fact that for better or for worse, in good times and in bad, the Alexian Brothers have been part of the history of Chicago for the past 150 years.

While the Brothers in Chicago had no psychiatric ward per se, there was always a section for "nervous and brain diseases" even in the 1870s. In the teaming melting pot that was Chicago of that era, there was plenty of disease of every variety, as well as, in a men-only hospital, alcoholism and other "social diseases" to which the human condition is heir. Care of the marginalized and the" outsider" was, and continues to be, a specific part of the Alexian mission, as it has been for centuries. Patients with mental disorders were both marginalized and outsiders, as a rule, especially if they were poor, much like today.

Still under the authority of the Aachen motherhouse in the 1880s, the rules were strict, conservative, and operated "after the German style" (Davidson 2012). The language of the hospital was German. Medical records were in German. The doctors spoke German, and the leadership was Aachen-trained. Because the Brothers did virtually every kind of work, from nursing to cooking to pharmacy to laundry, costs were low even for that time. In 1884, patient care cost the Brothers fifty-eight cents per patient per day. The average Brother's day lasted seventeen hours (including prayer), no one was paid, and the workweek was seven days. Sixty to 70 percent of the patients were charity, and the paying patients were paying about $3 to $5 per week. It was hard work, and slackers were not long tolerated.

The 1898 iteration of the Alexian Brothers Hospital on Belden Avenue was state-of-the-art for its day and had smaller, semiprivate two- and four-bed rooms. The nurses (and the cooks and the janitors and the launderers) were virtually all Alexian Brothers. In those days if a hospital wanted nurses it had to train them, and many hospitals had schools of nursing attached to and run by them. This was common well into the 1960s. When the Alexian training arm moved to Tennessee in 1938, the need for nurses became more acute, and the School of Nursing, heretofore training only Alexian Brothers, became open to laymen, one of only a few in the country accepting male nursing students. Male nurses were common in most European countries but for whatever reason were not accepted in England and the United States at the time. Student nurses served a function similar to medical interns and residents in the past (i.e., unpaid labor without which many hospitals would have found survival difficult).

In the days before health insurance, costs were always closely managed. At Catholic hospitals, costs were relatively low since even the fully trained nurses, if they were nuns or Brothers, were never paid. There were exceptions in Europe under the French after the secularizing sentiments (de-Christianization) of the French Revolution took control of religious institutions, and in a Prussianized Germany where the State did not always recognize or allow a vow of poverty. Under the American Constitution, the separation of church and state allowed no such intrusions by the state into religious matters so long as no civil laws were broken.[3]

Nurses and doctors in the days before World War II were akin to apprentices in the old trade or guild systems. They worked day and night for years, for room and board only. But in the end they could declare themselves trained, become licensed, and pursue independent practice.

---

[3] The most radical elements of the French Revolution wanted not only the de-Christianization of France, but the complete uprooting of every tradition guiding every aspect of traditional life. The week was changed to the ten-day week, so a month now contained three ten-day weeks. The names of days of the week, as well as months of the year, were changed to reflect this most radical transformation. Since the year 1789 reflected a Christian tradition regarding the birth of Christ some 1,789 years ago, 1789 was henceforth to be known as year one. As one can imagine, this new world was a bit much for many. Instead of getting one day off (Sunday) every seven days, workers didn't exactly relish the idea of a day of rest every ten days, whatever the name assigned to it. Radicalization eventually resulted in the Terror beginning in year five (1794), which resulted in the need to restore order, eventually leading to Napoleon.

After two years of hard labor, a nurse could get "registered" (i.e., licensed) as more states began to adopt licensure in nursing. To become a nurse, an undergraduate education was not necessary after high school. He or she learned what needed to be known on the job while performing essential nursing functions. Classroom instruction, when available, was a bonus but became more necessary as the scientific/technologic knowledge base expanded.

Medical training in nineteenth-century United States was often not much better except at the more prestigious schools, such as Johns Hopkins, where a German-style relationship among hospital, clinic, and university was established and scientific research encouraged. At least to become a nurse one had to do hands-on labor caring for the sick. In Chicago alone in the 1890s and early 1900s, there were more than forty medical schools of varying quality, longevity, and clinical exposure. It was possible to get a medical degree at some schools in the United States by attending a series of lectures and passing a few exams and seldom actually caring for a patient. Many medical schools were profit-making businesses (as more and more colleges are today), and for many schools the only admission criterion was ability to pay the tuition.

It was not until 1878 that the state of Illinois required doctors to actually graduate from a legitimate medical school in order to practice medicine in the state (Chicago Medical Society 1922). Oversight broke down in 1891 for blatantly political reasons (this is Illinois after all), and about twenty new, for-profit medical schools opened in the next decade. The internship came into existence as a period of clinical exposure so that the states could award licenses to doctors who had verifiably taken care of sick patients and passed a state exam. Each state had its own licensing exams, apparently suspicious of medical school quality, even though the graduate doctors had presumably already passed their medical school exams. The practice continues even today, although it has little to do with suspect medical school quality and more to do with political influence and control in its various forms.

In 1910, Abraham Flexner published the now-famous Flexner Report (Flexner 1910) on medical education in the United States and Canada. Flexner worked for the Carnegie Foundation and spent eighteen months visiting 155 medical schools and found dramatic differences among them. The better US schools like Johns Hopkins, Harvard, Northwestern, and the Universities of Michigan and Illinois were much like schools today, with two years of training in laboratory sciences followed by two years of clinical rotations in a teaching hospital. But many awarded medical degrees with far less, and Flexner's report lamented that "there is probably no other country in the world in which there is so great a distance and so fatal a difference between the best, the average, and the worst." The report specifically cited Chicago as the "plague spot of the country" because of the poor quality of many of its medical schools. The adoption of the recommendations of the Flexner Report for higher medical training standards lessened the dramatic discrepancies between the best and worst schools. It also dramatically reduced the number of medical schools and doctors graduating. Nonetheless, the legacy is that rather high-quality physicians can be found in the most rural or poverty-stricken areas of the country, albeit in lower numbers.

During the greatest part of the nineteenth century, the American public had no great interest in the quality of medical education. Compared to Europeans (and much of the rest of the world), Americans were bred on antiauthoritarianism and had an "anything goes" attitude about many issues, including medical practice. In time, however, the dramatic improvements in surgical outcomes, coupled with the dramatic lifesaving benefits of public health initiatives like vaccination and sanitation control, convinced the public of the value of science in medicine and demonstrated the worthlessness (and dangers) of many time-honored treatments, such as bleeding and purging.

As alluded to earlier, during the first half of the nineteenth century, most hospitals in the United States and elsewhere were little more than almshouses that provided care for the healthy indigent and the homeless, as well as the sick. In Chicago in 1832, essentially a wide-open frontier town, there was a cholera outbreak (an early example of a disease that starts in one corner of the world but, because of world travel and commercial contact, even then, spreads quickly to the whole planet; Chicago Medical Society 1922). By 1843, concern and fear prompted city leaders to build the first institution in the city devoted exclusively to medical care. Its purpose was to keep victims of contagious disease away from population centers. Later, in 1852, an attempt was made to segregate victims of smallpox from those of cholera.

With the exception of the large city clinics like those in Paris, Vienna,

Boston (Massachusetts General) and Baltimore (Johns Hopkins), the purpose of the vast majority of hospitals in this era was to protect the public, not necessarily to help the sick. This practice continued for victims of tuberculosis into the 1950s.

While the value of quarantine was known from the European experience with bubonic plague, and long before we understood how infections were caused and transmitted, the evolution of the hospital as a repository of high-tech medicine and applied biological science was to occur rapidly in the late nineteenth century. These changes occurred more rapidly in the practice of surgery and in public health than in other areas of medicine, where, for all practical purposes, most diseases were essentially untreatable.

In keeping with the more limited understanding in what we now refer to as psychiatric neuroscience, progress in psychiatry occurred slowly, if at all, despite attempts at biological research at various European universities and clinics. After 1900, a sense of therapeutic nihilism seemed to prevail, and it was indeed true that there was, in fact, no specific, reproducibly verifiable treatment for any major psychiatric condition. Psychoanalysis was just appearing on the world stage as a possible treatment for the less major conditions.

According to Kalinowsky (1984), the first successful biological treatment of any mental illness was in Vienna by Julius Wagner-Jauregg in 1917. Today we would not call neurosyphilis a mental illness exactly, but it produced psychiatric symptoms requiring long internments in mental hospitals. Significant improvement was observed in some patients during acute febrile episodes. Here the patient with neurosyphilis was injected intramuscularly with blood from humans infected with malaria and allowed to have ten to twelve fever bouts. The susceptibility of malaria to quinine allowed for the control (more or less) of the malaria. Meanwhile, the heat produced in the body by malaria proved lethal to the spirochetes infecting the brain and became an effective treatment until the advent of penicillin. Penicillin proved even more effective, as well as prophylactic, for neurosyphilis and its evil sibling, tabes dorsalis. Malaria treatment was only successful if the patient had syphilis and was obviously not directed at mental symptoms per se but at the underlying brain infection manifesting as psychiatric symptoms.

It's not that there wasn't anything going on in brain research. The

Germans were the first to encourage research in psychiatry. In Berlin in 1865, Wilhelm Griesinger joined the university, with its research ethic, to the psychiatric clinic and adopted the model later copied in the United States at Johns Hopkins. Alois Alzheimer described the syndromes of dementia now identified with his name. Studies of drugs and their effects on the nervous system, such as morphine for pain perception, were done. Research like Sigmund Freud's (1974) own early studies of cocaine, as topical anesthesia, as well as its effects on attention and cognition, was becoming commonplace. Shorter (1997) refers to the nineteenth century, in terms of psychiatry and neurology, as the German century.

During the nineteenth century, the French, for all their superiority in medicine in the first half of the century, took a regressive position when it came to psychiatry (Shorter). In France, political decisions decreed that research in psychiatry would occur in asylums and not, as in Germany, at the universities. Bénédict Augustin Morel popularized the concept of "degeneration," which was the belief that those with mental illnesses or mental retardation (or criminality or sexual deviations) would see succeeding generations create ever-increasing degrees of illness (Shorter). This belief was based on an erroneous evolutionary doctrine based on the French evolutionist Lamarck's theory of the inheritance of acquired characteristics. Even after Darwin's On the Origin of Species (1859), Lamarck's views still held considerable weight in France. This thinking led to the idea that what was anxiety in earlier generations could ultimately lead to dementia in succeeding generations. It also led to patients being labeled "degenerates," which explained the general population's abhorrence of the admission of mental illness or mental retardation in one's family.

However, the more limited understanding of psychiatric disorders in which a specific cause could not be identified manifested itself in a proliferation of schools of thought in psychiatry as the twentieth century dawned. From the French Revolution to about 1900, psychiatry seemed more and more firmly in the medical camp. After that time, and coincident with the rise of psychoanalysis and the apparent hopelessness in treating severe psychiatric disorders, it seemed less certain where psychiatry belonged.

Nevertheless, for the bulk of diseases commonly seen in general medical practice, there was not always a strong body of scientific evidence pointing clearly in one direction or another. As a result, various "schools" of healing developed in medicine, which gave rise to developments like osteopathy, chiropractic, naprapathy, homeopathy, and assorted spas, water cures, and "natural healing" theories of one kind and another, which persist into the present. This proliferation of "schools" in medicine reflected a lack of consensus on what constituted high-quality treatment and disease prevention even outside the psychiatric profession.

CHAPTER 4

Critical Developments in Surgery, Medicine, and Public Health

If prostitution is the oldest profession, certainly medicine is the second oldest. Throughout history I doubt that human beings in possession of prefrontal/frontal lobes (including Neanderthals), suffering any form of physical or mental malady, had any difficulty finding someone to treat it. The "public" has always demanded it, and any profession that is market driven is destined to succeed. No matter how primitive early bands of humans may have been, someone in their midst would've quickly come to the conclusion that he (or she) who offered answers and explanations (true or not) to natural phenomena and afflictions would exert great influence over their peers. By whatever names they were called, healers have always existed.

The only requirement was that they were convincing. No early human culture survived without these medicine men (shamans/priests/physicians), and since everything was a kind of magic, it didn't seem to occur to most human societies to even attempt to separate the supernatural from the mystical from what we would now refer to as "objective reality" or scientific proof. Nevertheless, with enough trial-and-error practice, many of these practitioners developed enough practical knowledge to be effective in relieving some human suffering. It apparently worked for thousands of years ... until it didn't.

It didn't work anymore, because major killers like bubonic plague, smallpox, and cholera did not respond to traditional folk medicine. Those who sought the methods of objective reality became more effective than those who didn't, and success is a powerful motivator. Historians called it the scientific revolution.

Although the nineteenth century saw the most incredible leaps in basic knowledge in the medical professions of any century before (and possibly since), in 1800, the gaps in knowledge between the various medical "specialties" were not that great. Even the use of the term "specialty" was generally not warranted. In America, someone like Benjamin Rush, psychiatrist and signer of the Declaration of Independence, we refer to as "psychiatrist," because he chose to work at the Institute of the Pennsylvania Hospital, which treated the mentally ill. Other than working there, there was probably little specific training that he received beyond his regular medical education (mostly by apprenticeship), as was the case for most, even university-trained physicians.

In some strange way it's curiously comforting to learn that college students in the 1830s and 1840s enjoyed getting "high" as much as their modern counterparts, throwing parties known as "ether frolics" on weekends and holidays (International College of Surgeons). Nitrous oxide, popularly known as "laughing gas," was also a big hit among partygoers. In December 1844, at an affair where audience members paid 25 cents to watch each other behave foolishly, a dentist, Horace Wells, discovered that a man injured during an intoxicated episode felt no pain despite significant injury. Wells contacted another dentist friend, William Morton, who decided to try nitrous oxide to extract a tooth. When the chemist (pharmacist) couldn't get nitrous oxide, he suggested ether instead (so called since 1730, though originally called "sweet oil of vitriol," discovered in 1540 by German botanist Valerius Cordus) as having many of the same qualities, especially narcosis. It worked well for tooth extraction. It helped make the public less fearful of dentists.

Morton then suggested that ether might be useful in surgery and convinced a surgeon at Massachusetts General, John Collins Warren, to try it on a surgical patient.

October 16, 1846, marked the beginning of an important component of the modern surgical era.[4] At that time, ether anesthesia played a pivotal role in rendering the operating room of the time (often a dining room table) considerably less noisy and eliminated the need for large men to hold down screaming patients who sometimes preferred suicide to surgery. The news spread rapidly everywhere, helped no doubt by the reality that no one held a patent on ether, which was discovered (and apparently available) three centuries earlier. It is impossible to underestimate the enormity of this discovery, which in a single moment elevated the practice of surgery from horror show to healing art.

Prior to approximately 1750, the surgeon was considered the inferior of the physicians in the profession since to become a physician (in Europe) one had to attend a university. In Great Britain at that time, the title of "Doctor" was given to physicians only. Surgeons, often trained as barbers or butchers, preferred the hands-on approach and were mostly apprenticed into their profession. In sixteenth-century Europe, if a patient needed surgery, the physician referred him to his barber. In 1540 England, King Henry VIII granted a charter, marking the founding of the Company of Barber Surgeons, which two hundred years later evolved into the Royal College of Surgeons (Porter 1997). Surgeons in Britain are still referred to as "Mister," a title retained based on the British fancy for "tradition," even though surgeons attend university now. Also, in eighteenth-century England, the surgeon John Hunter began the careful study of human anatomy and encouraged other surgeons to do the same. What seems obvious to us today was not always obvious then, but the practice of surgery was elevated by the careful study of anatomy.[5]

---

[4] According to an exhibit at the International Museum of Surgical Science at the International College of Surgeons in Chicago, Dr. Crawford W. Long of Georgia was the first to use ether for anesthesia but never made it public. Also, in Japan, Dr. Seishu Hanaoka, in 1806, used an oral anesthesia, Datura, for surgical procedures with some success.

[5] There is an exhibit at the Royal College of Surgeons in Edinburgh featuring Arthur Conan Doyle, creator of Sherlock Holmes, who was a graduate of the medical school at Edinburgh. The Holmes character was patterned after a professor Joseph Bell, who would amaze students with his ability to examine a patient physically, using absolutely no conversation, and by exam alone, describe the patient's profession, area of residence, habits both good and bad, and myriad other characteristics. In a very early talking film (circa 1929) available as part of the exhibit, Conan Doyle

In the days before anesthesia, surgery was mostly about amputating limbs or removing abscesses. The good surgeon was the fast surgeon. The application of accurate anatomical knowledge gained by studying anatomy on real (dead) human bodies, coupled with the practical need for speedy technique on patients anesthetized by opium and alcohol, allowed leg amputations to be accomplished in three to five minutes by the best surgeons of the time. Dominique Jean Larrey, chief surgeon in Napoleon's army, claimed that at the Battle of Borodino (1812) "I performed in the first 24 hours, about 200 (amputations)" (Porter 1997). The young Charles Darwin, sent to medical school at Edinburgh by his physician father, was so horrified by the practice of surgery in the 1820s that he dropped out of medical school and went to Cambridge to become a clergyman (since his physician father felt he wouldn't be much good at anything else). Most of us today regard his leaving medical school as a fortunate turn of events, as with Berlioz.

The established medical schools of the late eighteenth and early nineteenth centuries were slow to take up the practice of dissection since most religious thinking of the period saw human dissection as sacrilegious and a sinful violation of the dead. A kind of alternative medical school developed that sanctioned dissection but also, unfortunately, gave rise to "body snatching," a practice memorialized in Mary Shelley's 1818 novel (more so the 1931 film) Frankenstein. These cases represented an early example of how science and the marketplace supported one another. Science needed a product (dead bodies), and the "market" responded. Some citizens of the time appeared to be worth more dead than alive and were rendered thus by early entrepreneurs in the "medical supply" business. In the short term, the public was horrified. In the long term, however, most would agree that the public was ultimately served well by doctors who studied human anatomy. Some years later, the more mainstream medical schools also began teaching anatomy courses using real human (dead) bodies.

By the mid-1800s, refinements in germ theory were being developed in France by Louis Pasteur, who was employed by the agricultural industry to

---

describes his chagrin at having created Sherlock Holmes. It seemed that the public would not accept that Holmes was a fictional character, and even up to as late as 1929, when the interview film was made, he was inundated with requests for information about Holmes's whereabouts, ancestry, later life history, and multiple proposals of marriage.

study the process of spoiling (DuClaux 1920). His conclusions regarding the growth of unwanted organisms were applied to surgery in England by Joseph Lister, who reported that from 1861 to 1865, 45 to 50 percent of amputations on his male accident ward (and in American Civil War hospitals) died of sepsis (infection). In 1865, he instituted a form of antiseptic technique based on his understanding of Pasteur's work and by 1869 reported a drop in mortality rates to 15 percent. Unfortunately, in much of the world, including the United States, his work was largely ignored until decades later. His sterile surgical techniques came to be called "Listerism," now immortalized only in a popular antiseptic mouthwash called Listerine.

In most of the world at the time, surgical and traumatic wound infections seemed like part of the natural order of the universe that could not be changed. The cause was thought to be "bad air," referred to as "miasma," or perhaps by a phenomenon referred to as "spontaneous generation," whereby decaying or damaged tissue spontaneously gave rise to the growth of bacteria. Louis Pasteur demonstrated his assertion that "all life is from life" in his famous swan neck flask experiment (DuClaux 1920). In it he demonstrated that bacteria would not grow in a sterilized broth preparation unless the flasks were broken open, thereby exposing the broth to spore-containing dust particles. So ended the theory of spontaneous generation.

As noted earlier, Pasteur's study of microorganisms led him to study the process of spoiling in milk, beer, and wine, an early collaboration of science and the business/agricultural world in the service of both profits and good health. In 1862, he and Claude Bernard developed a process in which liquids were heated to kill the microorganisms, and the process became known as pasteurization.

Of the 650,000 deaths in the American Civil War, about two-thirds were the result of disease. Germs killed more soldiers than bullets did. There were also plenty of wound infections secondary to traumatic injuries, or the aftermath of amputations or other wound debridement, in the absence of an understanding of germ theory and the need for sterile technique. If 50 percent of Joseph Lister's amputees died in his London accident ward, soldiers in the field could hardly expect better. Nevertheless, living together in camps with thousands of rural folk recently thrown together in unsanitary conditions generated its own public health nightmare and accounted for the majority of deaths in the Civil War.

Published reports of significantly reduced postsurgical infection rates by Lister in England were quickly adopted in Germany by 1875. They were only slowly accepted in the United States despite reports suggesting much higher survival rates in major surgical procedures. These developments (i.e., anesthesia and sterile technique) eventually generated a revolution in the practice of surgery, which resulted in dramatically fewer deaths during and after surgery and increased the likelihood that surgeons might choose the operating room over the dining room. Indeed, it was their ability to understand and, at an early stage, adopt and improve upon these new developments in surgery that propelled the Mayo brothers from an obscure backwater in southern Minnesota to world prominence. They innovatively used, applied, and developed the cutting-edge surgical technology of their time in ways similar to contemporaries Thomas Edison and Henry Ford and, in more recent memory, Bill Gates and Steve Jobs.

The Mayo historian Helen Clapesattle (1941) reports that a tornado hit the vicinity of Rochester, Minnesota, on August 21, 1883, resulting in major damage to property along with considerable morbidity and mortality of its citizens. There was, of course, no hospital and no agreement about how the masses of injured should be cared for. One doctor ordered that all injury victims be given emetics, believing that somehow the broken bones, lacerations, soft tissue injuries, and concussions could be vomited back to good health. Medical school was not required for doctoring in those days, especially on the frontier. The dead and injured were brought to various locations around Rochester, such as hotels, lodging houses, public buildings, and a local convent parlor.

Nursing personnel were sorely needed, but few were available. Everyone helped out initially, but after the first day the injured and sick still required ongoing treatment. There were very few available to give their full time to the formidable nursing tasks still needed. The elder Dr. Mayo approached the Mother Superior of a convent of nuns who operated a local girls' school and asked for their help in devoting their full-time attention to nursing the injured. Since it was still summer, the nuns were available, and the Mayo boys gave a quick course on everything-you-need-to-know-about-trauma-nursing and sent them quickly into action. The nuns eventually became fairly good at these tasks, and since there was no local hospital and one seemed to be needed, the nuns eventually decided to build one if the Mayos agreed to use it.

The elder Dr. Mayo advised them against going ahead with a hospital, giving three reasons: the city was too small to support a hospital; it would cost too much; and there was little likelihood of its success.

The convent's Mother Superior decided to go ahead with it anyway, and the Mayos agreed to use it if it was built. That turned out to be lucky for the nuns, because when the hospital was completed, none of the other doctors in the community would use it. There were two reasons, according to Ms. Clapesattle: most were not Catholic and didn't like the idea of supporting anything Catholic, and more importantly, lacking another cataclysm like the one in August 1883, they didn't see a reason for one.

They didn't appreciate the importance of "Listerism" and the rising importance of skilled nursing, especially during and after major surgery. The Mayo brothers did, and the rest, as they say, is history since the Mayo Clinic became, first and last, a surgical mecca.

The key public health developments of the very late eighteenth century to the mid-nineteenth century were vaccination and the discovery of the role of bacteria in the spread of infection. As early as 1796, Edward Jenner had used cowpox to create a cross-immunity to smallpox. He published his results in a series of three papers, which first appeared in 1798. According to Dr. William Osler (1921), the Chinese were using vaccination for smallpox three hundred years earlier. Vaccination was revolutionary and, for the times, counterintuitive. One protected against an infectious agent by deliberately administering the very agent of infection to an otherwise healthy person or animal (or child). One wonders what kind of informed consent document was created for these first clinical trials.

Once one of the great mass killers of history, smallpox is now nowhere to be found on planet Earth (except, as reported recently, in US government refrigerators). Today it has become popular to blame vaccination for supposedly "new" problems, such as autism and ADHD, with very little evidence, forgetting the millions of deaths and disabilities (does anyone remember polio?) virtually unknown today. Preventing a disease is never as sexy as surgically intervening in one, but the results have been incredibly positive, if largely taken for granted of late. Indeed, an antivaccination movement seems to be developing in the United States today, giving rise to new outbreaks of previously controlled and rather deadly diseases, echoing Karl Marx's warning that those who are ignorant of history may be doomed to repeat it.

The years between 1830 and 1900 were probably the most seminal in medical history and set the table for what was to come in the twentieth century. The role of bacteria in the causation of disease was unknown in 1845. There was, of course, lots of speculation.

One of the leading medical centers in the world was in Vienna, Austria, once the glittering capital of the Habsburg Empire. It was well known that the Vienna General Hospital's First Obstetrical Clinic had an extremely high mortality rate from what was then called "childbed fever," currently known as gram-negative septicemia, still quite deadly today. Moreover, another clinic at the same institution run by midwives had a significantly lower mortality rate. At least they kept mortality data.

It appears that the Vienna General Hospital's First Obstetrical Clinic was situated right next to the anatomical dissecting room, human dissection by this time having become legitimate. Doctors unwilling to waste valuable time would do dissections while waiting to deliver babies and would go directly from the dissecting room to the delivery room. In mid-May 1847, Dr. Ignaz Semmelweis instituted the practice of handwashing with chlorinated lime solutions and demonstrated a drop in mortality rates from childbed fever of 90 percent (Osler 1921). In April 1847, the mortality rate was 18.3 percent. In June, the rate was 2.2 percent, in July 1.2 percent, and in August 1.9 percent. In the following year, it was 0 percent in two of twelve months. Absolutely astounding!

Unfortunately, no one outside of Dr. Semmelweis and his students noticed. He had no explanation for his findings, because the germ theory of infection had not yet been developed. Chlorinated lime solution was chosen because he believed that doctors and students carried "cadaverous particles" on their hands from the autopsy rooms located near the obstetrical clinic, and these solutions were known to eliminate the putrid smell of infected autopsy tissue. Perhaps the "poison" was being killed or neutralized in some way. He became certain that doctors were transmitting something from the autopsy room to the obstetrics clinic and instituted the practice of handwashing.

A disease at this time in history was considered caused by many different and unrelated factors. Each case was considered unrelated to another, and his insistence that childbed fever had only a single cause was considered extreme at the time and was essentially ignored and ridiculed by the local medical community.

Findings from autopsies of women who died from childbed fever showed variable and inconsistent results, fostering the common belief that this condition was not one but a variety of yet-to-be-identified diseases. The belief was that disease was spread by "bad air" known as miasmas or "unfavorable atmospheric-cosmic-terrestrial influences," which was the professional way of saying that they didn't have a clue.

Semmelweis died in 1865 in Budapest, only fourteen days after being committed to a mental asylum. Cause of death is reported as infection, rumored to be secondary to a beating by hospital "guards" (not an Alexian asylum obviously). At his death, few in the medical profession accepted his opinions. Later, when Louis Pasteur in France demonstrated the validity of germ theory, Semmelweis's views were finally accepted. When Joseph Lister applied the principles of germ theory to surgical practice, surgical safety took off.

Stories like that of Semmelweis, and his struggle for acceptance in the face of what appears to be medical intransigence in what turns out to be a miraculous and momentous discovery, needs to be seen in perspective. Dramatic stories like this one have popular appeal, and we like stories about how everyone laughed at so-and-so but how so-and-so got the last laugh. Hollywood likes to dramatize these stories since the "hero" in history and in myth seems less heroic unless he goes through a "trial" (e.g., "The Labors of Hercules") or period of suffering before earning hero status.

However, Semmelweis didn't publish anything on his findings until 1858, and his major work on childbed fever was not published until 1861. Prior to that, his students wrote letters and gave lectures to inform the medical world. His lack of understanding of the process of infection led him to posit ideas about poisonous "cadaverous particles," which were difficult to prove and made it easy for others to impugn his theory of causation, which was, in fact, wrong. His observations had substance, but his science was problematic. His ideas made more sense after Pasteur formulated the principles of "germ theory," which were unknown in his time. He himself didn't realize that he was talking about the transmission of living organisms from dissection room to delivery room. Because this would require an entirely new paradigm, which neither he nor his contemporaries were ready for, his ideas were not accepted. It probably didn't help that Semmelweis was emotionally volatile and got angry with those who disputed his ideas. When he started calling them "murderers," it did not help him win friends and influence (most especially) doctors.

In the mid-nineteenth century, Vienna was arguably the most advanced city on the planet (Paris was still very strong) when it came to medical innovation and scientific advance. If one strolls through the atrium at the medical school of the University of Vienna, one will witness endless rows of busts and statues memorializing the university's faculty and students, the names of whom have populated the textbooks of surgery and medicine for the last two hundred years. Among the multitude are names like Virchow, Billroth, Semmelweis, Meynert, Brucke, Helmholtz, and even Freud (although Freud's bust is quite tiny compared to some and strikes one as an afterthought, although there are clearly many more people on the planet who've heard of Freud compared to Virchow or Billroth). If any place on earth would be open to a new vision of disease, it was probably Vienna.

However, what one needs to understand is that there were/are legions of doctors all over the world making observations, reporting their findings, and drawing conclusions about the nature, causes, and cure of diseases who ultimately turn out to be dead wrong. This is the normal course of events, which continues unabated today. It is the reason that doctors tend to be conservative and require confirmation from different sources before embracing new ideas since the great majority will, ultimately, disappoint. You may have heard the story of the mother of a soldier (or sailor, marine, or airman) in World War II who woke up one night in a fright, feeling that her son had been killed, and it turned out to be true. One seldom hears stories about the thousands of other mothers who had the exact same experience, whose sons did not die, or at least did not die on that day. Doctors are well aware of the tendency in us all to over-interpret random events.

The introduction of anesthesia in surgery allowed for longer and more complex procedures that were impossible before 1846, which then required more training and experience for surgeons to undertake them. Once undertaken, it was like the discovery of a new land, with new discoveries of surgery's possibilities almost weekly. With the addition of "Listerism," postsurgical survival increased dramatically. An obvious corollary was that surgical procedures became necessarily more sophisticated and, therefore, more expensive, with hospitals slowly evolving into the repositories of high-tech procedures and scientific (evidence-based) medical practice that they are today. However disadvantageous a dining room table may be for performing surgery, there is no doubting the cost advantage.

One more public health accomplishment needs to be mentioned at this point, without which the greatest engineering project in the world could never have happened. It was a dramatic demonstration of the superiority of scientific observation over speculation and traditional thinking. In 1898, the United States went to war over the issue of Cuban independence.

According to David McCullough's (1977) The Path Between the Seas, for every American killed by Spanish bullets, thirteen died of disease, primarily yellow fever, malaria, and typhoid. These diseases were known to be tropical in origin and, like so many other presumably airborne diseases, felt to be related to vapors and gases generated by decaying tropical vegetation. In 1848, Dr. Josiah Clark Nott, a general practitioner in Mobile, Alabama, published a paper in the New Orleans Medical and Surgical Journal, claiming with some confidence that malaria and yellow fever were transmitted by insects, possibly mosquitoes, and that vapors and gases had nothing to do with it.

In 1854, French naturalist Lewis Beauperthuy, traveling in Venezuela, came to the same conclusion as an American professor of obstetrics, Dr. Alfred Freeman Africanus King, who recommended eradicating malaria from Washington by means of window screens, the draining of swamps and pools, and the destruction of insects by specially designed traps (McCullough 1977). As usual, few paid any attention at all.

In 1880, a French military doctor in Algeria described tiny crescent-shaped bodies in the blood cells of a patient with malaria and felt he'd described the offending agent in this deadly disease. He reported his findings in a letter to the Academie De Medicine in Paris and wrote a small monograph, but the "bad air" theory was dominant, and nothing happened as the French began their attempt at construction of the Panama Canal. By the time the French gave up the effort in 1889, estimates of up to twenty-five thousand workers and a great number of the cream of the French engineering profession died of yellow fever and malaria. Three-quarters of the workers in the French project were black persons from Jamaica and other Caribbean islands. Blacks were thought to have some natural (today we'd say "genetic" or "constitutional") protection from the ravages of tropical climate that whites lacked. This turned out to be untrue, and, as a percentage of the canal-zone population, blacks were actually overrepresented among those who died of these diseases, according to McCullough.

In 1889, Dr. Carlos Juan Finley of Cuba published his views in a Cuban medical journal on yellow fever and malaria as possibly mosquito-borne. Because of the very peculiar natural history of this particular species of mosquito, it was difficult to prove his theory, and it was ignored. When the Americans came to Cuba in 1898, the US Army's Dr. Walter Reed worked with Finley to prove not only that yellow fever was transmitted by a mosquito, but a very specific species of mosquito, stegomyia fasciata, and nothing else. By 1901, US Army physicians Walter Reed and William Gorgas managed to eradicate yellow fever in Havana.

In India, British doctor Ronald Ross identified the Anopheles genera of mosquito as the only known carriers of malaria and sleeping sickness. Mosquito netting, screens on windows, and drainage of swamps saved millions.

When the Americans took over from the French in the construction of the Panama Canal, William Gorgas was appointed chief medical officer. He knew what needed to be done but couldn't get the budget or the staff until the death toll started to soar, and attracting skilled workers to the "bad air" of the tropics became nearly impossible. He finally did get the resources he required, and yellow fever and malaria were virtually eradicated and the canal successfully completed. Medical science saved lives in dramatic fashion. The old ways simply didn't work. Even in psychiatry there was optimism in that some "causes" were identified to the extent that identification of infectious agents (like syphilis) could be determined and pathology could point to visible changes in brain tissue and function. Even if treatments were so far ineffective, identification of cause had, as with the study of infection, eventually led to useful treatment.

And so, with increasing medical knowledge came a need for better training of doctors and nurses. More training required more time and more expense. Specialization in medicine and nursing became more and more necessary. Hospitals were now becoming more than just places where the poor went to die. Good intentions were no longer good enough. The $5-per-week hospital bed was rapidly becoming a thing of the past.

CHAPTER 5

THE PSYCHIATRIC HOSPITAL

Psychiatric hospitals have been around for centuries, primarily referred to as "asylums," which literally means a safe place. What's in a name? The word "hospital" is a relatively modern term when it comes to psychiatric conditions, and it has come to imply active treatment. "Asylum" presently and historically has implied the specter of long-term maintenance where the mentally ill were cared for until they either died or somehow got better. Patients did get better in some cases, but the process was seldom very rapid, and six-, seven-, or ten-year (or lifetime) stays were not uncommon. Except for the very wealthy, their care was seen as the responsibility of the local community or the county and, later in history, the state. Historical Colonial Williamsburg in Virginia has as one of its quaint colonial buildings, of all things, a mental asylum with chains, stocks and all.

In the nineteenth century, physicians who cared for the mentally ill, especially those with legal problems, were referred to as "alienists," in reference to the patient population. The Random House Dictionary lists the following as a definition of the word "alien": "a person who has been estranged or excluded," which aptly describes many a mentally ill person. "Psychiatrist" is a relatively recent term.

Twenty-four hundred years ago, Hippocrates described the symptoms of several mental illnesses and identified them as medical problems worthy of the physician's attention, but for most of human history it's been the community that's decided who is and who is not insane. According to medical historian Roy Porter (1997), it was the family or the parish or the town that took responsibility. If they could not cope with or control the individual, then the local authorities resorted to jails, dungeons, or other correctional facilities, much like we do today. For example, the largest mental facility in Illinois is now the Cook County Jail.

These were generally not medical institutions. Bethlem, in London (from whence comes the synonym for chaos and disorder, "bedlam"), was primarily a religious or municipal charity (Porter). A physician may have looked in from time to time to "physick" a violent patient by purging or bleeding while under restraint, but these were infrequent before the waning years of the eighteenth century. Even the Alexian Brothers institutions in the sixteenth-century Netherlands were not very likely medical institutions per se, although their mission was to care for the sick.[6]

The educated, as well as the not-so-educated, general public today thinks of psychiatry and psychiatrists as relatively recent phenomena, perhaps an outgrowth of indolent modernism or liberal thinking gone awry. Sometimes a relative of a mentally ill person will start a conversation with "I don't believe in psychiatry" or "My husband (or father, or mother, or uncle ... or dog) doesn't believe in psychiatry." These indeed are peculiar statements. On better days, one interprets these statements as meaning a rejection of whatever methods they believe psychiatrists are likely to employ, too often imperfectly. On bad days, one thinks they mean they doubt the existence of psychiatric disorders per se, or at least in their relatives.

As an undergraduate between 1958 and 1961, I was surprised to learn that one of every two hospital beds in the United States was occupied by a psychiatric patient. In chapter 1, we saw that in 1955 there were 560,000 state-supported psychiatric beds, and that figure did not include private psychiatric hospitals. Those figures must seem rather implausible to someone raised in more recent times. The reality is that mental illness is not a myth contrived by psychiatrists and other "establishment" (a popular term used in the sixties as a synonym for oppressive or reactionary) cronies designed to incarcerate those poor souls who would dare to be different. This was a popular 1960s perception, which still has fervent adherents. Psychiatry is definitely not a recent trend or fad, although treatments in

---

[6] The Alexian Brothers facilities in Germany to this day see work as rehabilitative and therapeutic and operate a number of businesses to which patients contribute and gain real work experience. These include an upscale hotel, a tree and plant nursery, an art gallery, and other work-training activities.

psychiatry, as well as other branches of medicine or surgery, can be trendy or faddish and always have been to some extent, present day included.

The American Psychiatric Association, officially founded in 1844, is the oldest continuously operating national medical society in the United States (the American Medical Association started in 1847), and a psychiatrist, Benjamin Rush, was the only physician signer of the US Declaration of Independence in 1776. Psychiatrists are not creations of affluence, and Sigmund Freud was not the first psychiatrist. He wasn't even a psychiatrist (by training) and spent little, if any, time studying psychotic patients, although his name came to be synonymous with the profession for many years.

Developments in Europe, as usual, had significant influence on psychiatric practice in America. The egalitarian ideals of the French Revolution no doubt played a role when Dr. Philippe Pinel famously "removed the chains" from the mentally ill at Paris's Salpêtrière (females) and Bicêtre (males) asylums and adopted a more humane model of mental treatment (Porter 1997). He didn't exactly walk in on a Tuesday and remove all the chains by Wednesday, but Pinel, a devout Catholic who wanted to become a priest at first, believed that the mad behaved like animals because they were treated like animals. He was gradually able to institute a policy of nonrestraint for a majority of patients. As the French Revolution gained momentum, Frenchmen soon learned that the unchained mentally ill were going to be the least of their problems.

The English version of Pinel was the Quaker William Tuke, who introduced his version called "Moral Treatment" (Porter). His version dictated treatment in a bucolic location away from the din of the city, in quiet comfort, where one's "nerves" could heal. His version seemed to work much better for patients than at Bethlem in London. Eventually these ideas crossed the Atlantic.

In 1811, the Massachusetts legislature granted a charter to the Massachusetts General Hospital Corporation (Little 1972). The intent from the outset was to treat both mental as well as physical illnesses. From day one there was to be a general medical, along with a psychiatric, brick-and-mortar facility. The first psychiatric patient was admitted on October 1, 1818. The principles of "Moral Treatment" were implemented. At the time it was only the fourth hospital in the United States designed for the treatment of the mentally ill. By 1844, there were thirteen such hospitals on the Eastern Seaboard. In that year, the thirteen superintendents of the thirteen hospitals got together and founded the Association of Medical Superintendents of American Institutions for the Insane. Later it was renamed the American Psychiatric Association, referred to earlier.

In 1826, a wealthy Boston merchant, John McLean, bequeathed almost $120,000 (a grand sum at the time) to the Massachusetts General Hospital's psychiatric division, and its name was changed to The McLean Asylum for the Insane, today's McLean Hospital in Belmont, Massachusetts.

In 1882, McLean Hospital established the first school of psychiatric nursing in the United States and, in 1888, the first basic and clinical laboratories to study biological factors in mental illness. As was the case with most mental hospitals needing to support long periods of confinement, McLean was self-sustaining to as late as 1944. Most food was produced on its own farm, and it operated a blacksmith and an upholstery shop. Up until at least 1944, work was considered a therapeutic intervention and not a form of patient abuse.

Social reformers in the United States, like Dorothea Dix, admired the "asylum in the country" model and successfully lobbied the states to build many. The giant state hospitals for the mentally ill came into being and became huge institutions, which proved long on isolation and short on rehabilitation. With sometimes many thousands in residence, the worthy goals of moral treatment were either lost or greatly reduced. The mega–mental hospitals of the past are no more, which has been taken to be a good thing, though good only when humane alternatives are developed for chronic patients still in need of care. Hospitals are still preferred to prisons if there's a choice.

Closer to home, the Alexian Brothers of Chicago was incorporated in March 1869 with the purpose of "establishing and conducting hospitals, the nursing of sick male persons, and the nursing and taking care of idiots and lunatics of the male sex" (Davidson 1990). (Today we consider some of these terms to be at least politically incorrect if not downright offensive. Like everything in nature, language and words evolve over time).

In Chicago there was not a specific psychiatric ward, but the 1884 annual report shows that they cared for three patients with "melancholia" and a patient with "acute mania" in the section of the report titled "Diseases of the Nervous System," which also included migraine, alcoholism, meningitis, and idiocy.

The Alexian Brothers in St. Louis opened their first hospital in February 1870, and when they built a larger hospital in 1874, it came with a detached building that claimed a "70 foot veranda, which had no (direct) connection with the main hospital, where the unfortunate nervous patients were cared for" (Dahl 2012). The Alexian hospital in St. Louis was the first in that city to have a separate psychiatric division and treat alcoholism and mental illness as diseases, the German model of psychiatric illness. In 1879, $300 was allocated for alterations to the detached building. This appeared to be an attempt to set up the detached building as an "asylum" for the long-term care of the chronic mentally ill. Patients requiring only short-term care were housed on the fourth and fifth floors of the main hospital. Even at this time in history, there was official acknowledgment at Alexian hospitals that psychiatric disorders came in both acute and chronic forms. This has very likely been evident ever since the development of settled civilizations.

The 1973 film The Exorcist was a dramatized portrayal of an actual exorcism, which reportedly took place in 1949 on the fifth floor of the St. Louis hospital. Records indicate clearly that psychiatry was part of the general hospital's everyday operation. The doctors apparently were not averse (or were not recorded as averse) to what are now referred to as "alternative therapies," this despite the Alexians' traditional preference for the medical over the theological model. Perhaps it was what today we'd refer to as a "patient preference."

With respect to psychiatric facilities in Chicago, admittedly a frontier town in the 1840s, it is reported that there was a private "retreat" somewhere north of North Avenue as early as 1847, but no records apparently have survived (Dahl). In 1854, Cook County moved its almshouses to a site known as "Dunning," where an asylum was one of the buildings. This was known as the Cook County Hospital for the insane. In 1912, the state of Illinois took over its operation, and it became the Chicago State Hospital, or "Dunning," as it was usually referred to by the locals.

Treatment in the early years of the twentieth century was largely custodial since there was no known truly effective medical treatment for any major mental illness. Some did recover, and Tuke's "Moral Treatment" showed the value of humane care alone. Chicago State became an enormous facility and probably did little for property values in the area, although it was there before most of the houses as the expanding city grew around it. For those who grew up on the streets of Chicago's inner city, Chicago State Hospital seemed to symbolize despair and hopelessness. Its residents, sometimes visible to citizens of the city through its tall fences and gates, epitomized "crazy" in the popular imagination, including my own. Looking at the sheer size of this hospital in the 1940s and 1950s, covering perhaps one hundred acres plus with multiple buildings, one could easily imagine that 50 percent of all hospital beds in the country were psychiatric.

CHAPTER 6

TWENTIETH-CENTURY MEDICAL INTERVENTIONS IN PSYCHIATRY BEFORE DRUGS

During the nineteenth century, considerable research was devoted to psychiatry, especially in German-speaking countries, and a multitude of discoveries of great scientific merit were made. Since psychiatry and neurology were part of the same investigative process, in the medical world there was little difference in training and patients treated. Those neurologists who chose to work in psychiatric hospitals, or more exclusively with psychiatric patients, became identified as psychiatrists (e.g., the neurologist Sigmund Freud) or alienists.

The research of Dr. Alois Alzheimer led to the identification of the most common form of dementias now identified with his name. There were investigations into the effects of various drugs in the brain, like the pain-relieving and addictive properties of morphine. Sigmund Freud (1974) investigated the various cognitive and anesthetic properties of cocaine. The specific cause (the treponema spirochete) of the psychiatric symptoms seen in syphilis of the brain (neurosyphilis) was identified. Other causes of brain pathology that affected behavior and cognition were identified, but in the majority of psychiatric conditions seen in hospital and clinic, specific causes or underlying pathophysiologies were impossible to identify given the scientific technologies of the era.

This led to a sense of therapeutic nihilism in psychiatry and started a movement toward other ways of explaining psychiatric symptoms and their causation. As you will see in chapter 9, even Sigmund Freud was put off by severely ill psychiatric patients, generally considered untreatable and hopelessly chronic. As Kalinowsky (1984) writes,

> it seemed more sophisticated to concern oneself with the psychodynamics of psychopathological phenomena than with primitive physical treatments. I therefore switched to the psychoanalytical approach of Paul Schilder. Schilder's historical importance was that he was the first to recognize that psychological and biological concepts do not exclude each other.

According to Kalinowsky (1984), in 1917, Julius Wagner-Jauregg, at the Psychiatric University hospital in Vienna, conducted the first successful medical treatment for any mental illness in modern medical history.[7] It was based on the observation (this being still the heyday of observational medicine) that certain psychotic patients improved significantly during and shortly after febrile episodes. Because malaria was relatively controllable with quinine, blood from malaria patients was injected into patients who had general paresis (infections of the brain with the syphilis spirochete) and allowed to have ten to twelve fever bouts. Of the nine patients reported on in his initial report, three appeared to have been cured entirely, three were improved but still ill, and three were unchanged (The Rule of Thirds, well known among medical students and beyond). From then until the advent of penicillin more than twenty years later, this remained the treatment of choice for neurosyphilis. Apparently the intense body heat was lethal to the treponema spirochete in the brain. Although today we would not say that neurosyphilis is a mental illness per se, and this treatment did not prove useful in schizophrenia or other psychiatric disorders, it did arouse

---

[7] If Medicine is in fact the 2nd oldest profession, then one would have to believe that the Egyptians, Babylonians, Chinese, and Greeks certainly had their "cures," but outcome data, for what conditions, are unavailable. What we know for sure is that all cultures certainly had treatments for everything (their public would've demanded it, just like today), but it's also likely that distinctions between mental and physical disorders were not usually recognized or were very porous.

the hope that the investigation of agents that influence the brain was worth pursuing. It helped dispel the therapeutic nihilism of the time, according to Kalinowsky.

Insulin was isolated in the 1920s and found its way into psychiatric treatment (Kalinowsky). It was in general use, in small doses, as a sedative and to "build up" and increase appetite in hospitalized patients. Again, at the psychiatric university hospital in Vienna, Manfred Sakel made use of the observation that a few schizophrenic patients responded to the very small doses of insulin given for "build up" by going into a hypoglycemic (low blood sugar) coma. These patients were obviously hypersensitive to small doses of insulin. When they awoke they appeared to be greatly improved for a time before relapsing. Sakel then decided to explore insulin as a specific treatment in its own right under controlled conditions, instead of by accident, since there was no other viable treatment for these chronic patients.

In 1933, it was considered by many to be the most effective treatment for schizophrenia before the advent of antipsychotic medications in the 1950s. However, it was expensive and time-consuming in that it was an all-day procedure. It required a team of highly trained professionals to be conducted safely and needed repeated sessions over time. As a result of "insulin shock" therapy (the low blood sugar sometimes resulted in a seizure, but improvement did not require a convulsion), some chronic schizophrenic patients got significantly better, pointing the way toward a need for rehabilitation post treatment. The possibility of improvement led to more research on prognostic factors in schizophrenia. The development of various clinical and social measures of improvement followed, which heretofore had not seemed necessary since they were considered hopeless anyway.

Two other developments in the 1930s proved important for the psychiatry practiced in hospital settings. One was the development of convulsive therapies, especially electroconvulsive therapy (ECT). The other was leucotomy (lobotomy). Both were originally focused on the treatment of schizophrenia since schizophrenics represented the largest population of chronic patients found in the psychiatric hospitals of the time. It's important to keep in mind that, for the vast majority of very ill psychiatric patients, there was no effective treatment available, which is why physicians pursued their clues where they found them.

The development of convulsive therapies began about 1934 with

Dr. Ladislas von Meduna, a Hungarian psychiatrist at the University of Budapest. There was an unproven but generally accepted belief at the time that epilepsy and schizophrenia were somehow antithetical or in some strange way incompatible. In those patients where schizophrenia and epilepsy did coexist, it was a clinical belief that, after a seizure, patients seemed to improve, at least for a time. Dr. Meduna looked for a way to explore this clinical impression by inducing seizures deliberately under controlled conditions. He used oil of camphor inhalation in his first five cases[8] and then switched to cardiazol (Metrazol), which could be used intravenously for better control. There was enough observable improvement to warrant continued investigations, and knowledge of his work spread.

Meanwhile at the University of Rome, Ugo Cerletti and Lucino Bini began experimenting with the possibility of inducing seizures electrically (Kalinowsky). Drugs took variable periods of time to induce the seizure and were less precise and less predictable. Electrical administration induced seizures immediately. After several years experimenting on pigs at a local Roman slaughterhouse (slaughterhouses were using electrical stimulation to render pigs unconscious prior to the actual slaughtering), they treated their first patient in March 1938 using the technique we now refer to as "unmodified" ECT. Unmodified ECT consisted of an electrical stimulus to the brain through electrodes placed on both sides of the forehead just in front of the ears. Since this is where the temporal lobes of the brain are located, the placement became known as "bitemporal." No anesthesia or muscle relaxants were used, but the seizure itself rendered the patient unconscious. Unfortunately, side effects did occur with occasional fractures related to tightly contracting muscles and periods of apnea (loss of respiratory activity) during the seizure itself, which averaged about thirty seconds but could go longer. Lack of respiratory activity reduces oxygen flow to the brain, which,

---

[8] There was actually precedent in the medical literature for the use of convulsive therapy. The *London Medical Journal*, in 1785, published the case of a mental patient "seized with mania with few intervals of reason." The physician, Dr. C. Oliver, for some unexplained reason gave camphor inhalations to this patient, and fifteen minutes later he had an obvious convulsive seizure. He was reportedly normal for some unspecified period of time and then relapsed. Two years later, he was again given camphor with the same result. Again, his behavior and personality normalized, but when sent home he relapsed again.

if extended, could result in damage. A seizure greatly increases the oxygen requirements of brain cells. Modified ECT came later.

ECT was first used in the United States in 1940 through several Italian psychiatrists who had migrated here at about that time. Like every new and potentially effective treatment in psychiatry or general medicine, it quickly gets used in conditions other than schizophrenia. In that way, a few years later, Dr. A. E. Bennett in the United States reported that while ECT was sometimes effective in cases of schizophrenia, it could at times be remarkably beneficial in depression and mania. These "affective disorders" (depression and mania) remain ECT's primary indications after the failure of adequate response with psychotherapy and multiple medications.

Because of side effects, A. E. Bennett also began explorations into what we now refer to as "modified" ECT (Kalinowsky). Bennett's research showed the most egregious complications of ECT—fractures related to intense muscle contractions—could be eliminated by using a muscle relaxant. He first used curare, but later the much safer succinylcholine eliminated fractures completely as an issue in ECT. Today stimulators use micro doses of electricity compared to what Cerletti and Bini were using. Complications other than short-term memory loss are now rare. Today all ECT is administered with both muscle relaxants and general anesthesia, with continuous oxygen infusion and respiratory support throughout the procedure. Those who oppose any biological treatment in psychiatry will often show a film of patients receiving unmodified ECT as an example of psychiatric barbarism. The difference can be compared to the experience of surgery before and after the introduction of general anesthesia except that ECT is infinitely less dangerous.

Leucotomy (lobotomy) is sometimes spoken of as the twentieth-century Frankenstein story (often mentioned in the same sentence with ECT), with the Portuguese Dr. António Egas Moniz and American Walter Freeman alternately playing the title role. In order to do justice to this history, I beg indulgence on your part to allow a small digression with the promise of returning quickly to the topic under discussion.

Frankenstein is the 1818 novel by Mary Shelley, who was the second wife of the English romantic poet Percy Bysshe Shelley. The Romantic age was the period in European and American history comprising the first fifty years or so of the nineteenth century, following immediately after the age of reason in the eighteenth century. The Age of Reason promised that the study of nature (what we now call science) would lead mankind into a marvelous new order. All diseases would be stamped out or at least greatly ameliorated, and citizens (as opposed to subjects) would be rid of their kings and nobles. More just and prosperous societies would soon follow.

Surprise! It didn't exactly happen that way. Expectations and hopes were well beyond what reason (science) and the available technologies of the time were able to deliver. By 1800, people were still getting sick and dying, the enlightened French were still decapitating (albeit at a lesser rate) "enemies of the state," and Napoleon, the symbol of revolutionary righteousness and champion of the common man, gave himself the very unrevolutionary title of emperor. Idealistic intellectuals became disillusioned, and reaction set in. Reason had presumably not delivered on its alleged promises. Violence and social disorganization followed, and folks began to long for the good old days. Since reason (science) hadn't paid off quickly enough, maybe a more "romantic" re-vision of the past would.

Such was the state of things when, in 1816, Lord Byron, Percy Shelley, Mary Shelley, and John Polidoro, looking for something to do in the cold of winter at Byron's villa in Switzerland, challenged one another to see who could write the best horror story. Polidoro eventually came up with The Vampyre, and Mary wrote Frankenstein. Novels in those days often had alternative subtitles (to enlighten dull readers?), and Mary's full title was Frankenstein, or The New Prometheus.[9]

In the novel, Victor Frankenstein is taught from childhood to study

---

[9] Prometheus was a Greek god who had an unusual sympathy for mankind and, depending on the source, either had something to do with creating humankind or at least became our greatest benefactor. He was a rebellious sort. He often found himself protecting or otherwise backing humans and enraging the chief god, Zeus, who didn't particularly like mortals. In defiance of the will of Zeus, Prometheus stole fire (equated in Greek mythology with civilization) from Mt. Olympus and gave knowledge of it back to man, along with other trappings of civilization, such as knowledge of writing, mathematics, agriculture, and medicine. As punishment, Prometheus was bound to a rock with an eagle chewing on his liver, which would regenerate overnight and be chewed again the following day. As punishment for man, Zeus created woman. The first woman was named Pandora, who was not a nice lady and from whose jar (not a box) was unleashed disease, pestilence, war, and other evils plaguing civilization then and now. The ancient Greeks were a tad misogynistic.

science as a way to better humanity. What he ends up creating is an eight-foot-tall, rather grotesque figure with an anger management problem. Dr. Frankenstein's creation basically has a good heart deep down but is not well received by the humans whom he encounters. Although the novel is very different from the film version, the outcome is the same; science is practiced by madmen with an excess of hubris who will ultimately do more harm than good. This is why Prometheus was bound and why Adam and Eve (who bit into an apple from the tree of knowledge) were expelled from the Garden of Eden. Humans who aspire to the knowledge of the gods are destined by fate to ignominious failure.

So who was António Egas Moniz? He was a Portuguese neurologist who studied and taught neurology in Paris before becoming professor of neurology at the University of Lisbon. In 1927, he did the first-ever (reported) cerebral angiography, a procedure still commonly used today, which has turned out to be of significant benefit to mankind. He hoped for a Nobel Prize for his work, but it didn't happen. Moniz was probably not a neurological adventurer but someone who studied carefully the risks and benefits he subjected his patients to. Cerebral angiography is not an innocuous procedure even today and certainly not in 1927, when a safety profile had yet to be established. The issue, of course, is, as with all medical/surgical procedures, did the benefits outweigh the risks, and how does one go about determining that?

In the 1930s, as well as today, the frontal and prefrontal lobes were thought to play an important role in the kind of thinking impairments or logical errors seen in schizophrenia. The following textbook example is often given: "The president's name is Barack. My name is Barack. Therefore, I must be the president." There were also mood components resulting in fear, terror, and sometimes-violent behavior seen by these patients as self-defense.

However, the stimulus for Moniz to think of leucotomy (leuco = "white" in Greek, referring to the white matter tracts of the brain) as a viable possibility in the treatment of mental illness reportedly came during a lecture he attended given by two American physiologists. Carlyle Jacobsen and John Fulton were in Rome to report on the behavioral effects of removal of the frontal lobes in aggressive primates. You may recall our discussion in chapter 4 that mental institutions could be dangerous places (whence comes the term "bedlam") for both staff and patients, which is why restraints, straitjackets, and wet packs were in use. The lecture presumably gave Moniz the idea that possibly, by "disconnecting" the prefrontal areas from the rest of the brain by cutting (initially done by injecting pure alcohol) the white matter corticothalamic tracts, some of the more violent symptoms in various mental disorders might be ameliorated. This, he hoped, might allow for discharge in otherwise chronically institutionalized patients.

Moniz did not claim that the procedure was going to cure mental illnesses or that there would not be undesirable sequellae. Neurosurgical procedures of the time had attained a degree of precision, but more exact stereotactic techniques were not fully developed, and absolute precision was difficult to achieve. The goal was to relieve the suffering of patients who had spent many years in long-term institutional care and believed that the available evidence was that the benefit (relief of suffering and agitation) outweighed the potential, still relatively unknown negatives. His goal was to treat the most severe and most chronic of the mentally ill and provide some relief. His work was careful enough, and various publications on the procedure credible enough, that a Nobel committee in 1949 awarded him a share of the Nobel Prize in Medicine and Physiology for his introduction of leucotomy. The fact that he had earlier developed cerebral angiography and did not get a Nobel may have played a role. When in later years Moniz was being compared to Dr. Frankenstein by many psychiatrists, the Nobel committee was requested to invalidate his prize. The committee refused, believing that the evidence of positives outweighed the evidence of negatives. That controversy is still being debated.

Moniz apparently did not do long-term follow-up of the cases he and neurosurgeon Pedro Almeida Lima operated upon. This was a major failing since there turned out to be long-term negatives in numbers of patients not always apparent early. There was some oversight, but the apparent hopelessness and chronicity of the patients led to a hope that the potential benefits would outweigh the negatives.

However, when the procedure came to the United States, neurologist Walter Freeman, who worked with the neurosurgeon James Watts, enthusiastically took it up. They did their first cases in 1936, almost immediately after learning of Moniz's work. These were done in hospitals and as carefully as James Watts could perform them. In recent years, brain surgery has become synonymous with precision and accuracy in the popular imagination, and with good reason given the sophistication of current imaging and stereotactic technologies. The brain is a relatively small organ packed with myriad anatomically different cell types, and its complexity is orders of magnitude beyond other organs in the body. It is the site of all human emotion, cognition, perception, abstractness, and creative thought. Somehow the brain creates the "mind."

But in the 1940s, in the absence of stereotactic precision, they were often cutting more than "just" (not to imply these are trivial) white matter tracts. They were in effect cutting blindly to some extent.

In 1941, Freeman and Watts operated on Rosemary Kennedy, who was only twenty-three at the time. Depending on what one reads, Rosemary was "almost" normal intellectually prior to her leucotomy and afterward was unable to walk or talk coherently and institutionalized for the rest of her life in a kind of vegetative state (Kessler 1996). According to one report, Rosemary had changed from a well-behaved teen to a rebellious and uncontrollable young adult, and her father, Joseph P. Kennedy, who had major ambitions for his children, felt that Rosemary was going to embarrass the family (Leamer 1994). Since other interventions had apparently failed (whatever they were), her father contacted Dr. Freeman and had a lobotomy performed on Rosemary, allegedly without telling her mother. This case report is often used as an example of patient abuse at its worst and the horrible outcomes in lobotomy.

It is, in fact, no example at all but a combination of a few facts, lots of rumors, with information flow controlled tightly by the family. Disabilities in those times were a major source of embarrassment, of which the physical disability of Franklin Roosevelt was a good example. He couldn't walk unaided, but in newsreels he's always seen standing as if "normal." In the case of Rosemary, it was impossible to assess her intellectual state pre- and postsurgery, because the family did everything they could to hide whatever her disabilities were in the first place. In boarding school at age fifteen, she was isolated from her peers and taught individually by two nuns. She was estimated to have an IQ in the sixties before surgery, although some have disputed that since she's alleged to have been something of an accomplished letter writer (Leamer). It was later reported that at least some (most likely all) of her letters to organizations and persons were written by others and carefully copied by Rosemary (Leamer 1992; Collier and Horowitz 1984). The press was never allowed to interview her, but she was, at one time, alleged to be working as a kind of special education teacher. She has since been often referred to as "retarded," and the Kennedys' support of organizations for the developmentally disabled is well known. Some allege that the retardation was related to the lobotomy, but this is highly unlikely.

However, lobotomy was never said to be a treatment for mental retardation, and the clear implication was some form of mental illness. Political feelings about the Kennedy family—and Joseph P., in particular—colored everything associated with the story, giving support to one theory that Joseph P. was simply embarrassed by Rosemary's behavior and had her lobotomized to shut her up. As a story about lobotomy, this one has little value except for the interview granted by James Watts himself after Rosemary died in 2005. It shows just how imprecise the procedure was. Watts said that after making bilateral (for right and left hemisphere access) incisions, and the patient awake (the brain itself has no pain sensors) using only a mild tranquillizer, Freeman guided the extent of Watts's cutting by asking questions and talking to Rosemary. They stopped when she allegedly became incoherent. These procedures were rather inexact (i.e., they could not precisely isolate what was being cut).

In 1947, Freeman decided to "improve" on Moniz's procedure and the one used by himself and Dr. Watts. He eventually developed a less precise but much more cost-effective and rapid procedure, which later became known as transorbital leucotomy or the "ice pick" approach. Using this technique (literally a sterilized ice pick), Freeman felt he could dispense with hospitals, and leucotomy became an office procedure, which could be done at state hospitals with limited budgets. He approached the brain bilaterally through its thinnest part just above the eyes at the cranial floor. He hit the blunt end of the ice pick with a hammer, which got him through the thin bone at the base of the brain below the prefrontal cortex. He then made wide swaths, severing not only the white tracts but also swaths of gray matter indiscriminately. Freeman published, spoke widely about, and reported remarkable results with few serious side effects. James Watts felt that this new procedure was an outrage and separated himself from Freeman in 1947, after which Freeman did the procedures himself. When criticisms mounted on the East Coast, Freeman moved to California and began doing his procedure for virtually anyone who asked. Lobotomies were reported to have been used against their will, on violent criminals, homosexuals, and other "undesirables." Some of this was rumor, but some may have been factual.

According to the 2008 PBS documentary in the American Experience series "The Lobotomist," Freeman sidestepped the usual peer-reviewed channels and went directly to the press, who, then as now, love stories of dramatic cures and courageous pioneers. Freeman (according to this documentary) did nineteen procedures on persons under eighteen years old and one on a four-year-old! He began to do lobotomies for any and all manner of mental affliction and allegedly even for what is now referred to as ADHD. All these were without oversight or careful follow-up and with what were believed to be very negative consequences for many. When he was heckled at a psychiatric meeting, he produced a large stack of letters from patients and families thanking him for the help he gave them, some of which were shown on the PBS program, along with a live patient and daughter who felt they'd been helped significantly. Freeman eventually went on a long journey across the country to look up and report on as many of his operated patients as possible (Freeman 1957).

According to this PBS program, he did a total of 2,900 procedures between 1939 and 1967, when he lost his hospital privileges after the death of a patient. Lobotomy turned out to be the Frankenstein story, twentieth-century edition, at least in the United States. But until the advent of the first antipsychotic drug in 1954, lobotomies were still done in the United States at Massachusetts General, the Mayo Clinic, and elsewhere across the globe, presumably with greater care and precision. When the antipsychotic drugs began to appear in the 1950s, they were often referred to as "chemical lobotomy," meaning same effect, different means, but lobotomies came to an abrupt end. The term "lobotomy" became equated with the term (suggested by Freeman) "psychosurgery," and both words became infamous.

So was there any merit at all in the context of this otherwise very controversial story? The answer here turns on the issue of whether the patients were better or worse off in the final analysis, given what their lives had been up to at the point of surgery. In order to rationally evaluate these kinds of data, it's important to find credible, objective follow-up. At this point I believe we should look at some long-term follow-up studies since only by studying the outcomes of the patients operated upon can the merit question be addressed. One can agree, however, that operating on the brain of a misbehaving four-year-old is difficult to justify, no matter how ardently a frazzled parent may lobby for it.

Miller (1967) at the University of Toronto reported on a follow-up of 116 cases in 1967 of patients operated on from 1948 to 1952. This was a prospective study. In a prospective study the protocols and parameters are worked out prior to surgical intervention. Patients were evaluated pre- and postsurgery using point rating scales developed for this study. Using these scales, patients were seen by the researchers at six months, one year, two years, four years, five years, and ten years after surgery. The average time ill was 9.4 years, and the average time in the hospital was five years. The surgical procedure was carefully detailed and used, as exactly as possible, on all patients. Seventy-three percent of patients were schizophrenic, 19 percent affective psychoses, and the rest severe, hospitalized anxiety disorders. Before being selected for surgery they were presented before a selection board, and criteria for surgery were evaluated. Social functioning at these various review points was evaluated with information from family, social agencies, and hospital personnel for those in the hospital when evaluated. This was a professional research design looking at all aspects of patient functioning. Many find these kinds of studies tedious and not exciting to the media, but this is the way this clinical research needed to be done.

Results were: 67 percent of those operated on were able, after surgery, to live outside of a hospital, mostly permanently; 26 percent had periodic relapses, but these were temporary; 75 percent were able to work productively; and 38 percent of these were able to do high-caliber productive work. Of the 33 percent who were not out of the hospital, most were deemed better but still dependent on the hospital. However, 6 percent developed seizures (usually controlled by anticonvulsants), and 91 percent showed evidence of at least some "personality defect." There are personality defects reported with leucotomy variously characterized as disinhibiting, silly, or lacking concern with social convention. However, many of these patients were schizophrenics, and personality deficits are often reported in schizophrenic patients in various stages of recovery who have not undergone leucotomy. Weight gain was common. Two percent died as a result of complications related to the surgery. Nevertheless, based on their report, in some cases of very intractable illness, they felt that the benefits outweighed the negatives, and these researchers felt there was a case for the procedure in carefully selected patients.

In another study, Sloke and Gilder (1968) reported in The Journal of the American Medical Association on a follow-up of twenty-seven private but very chronic (prior to surgery) patients of psychiatrists at Washington University, St Louis. Between 1951 and 1959, they used a variation on the classic technique. Private patients were used since follow-up by the same doctors was possible over many years. In twenty-five of these twenty-seven patients, the leucotomy was unilateral on the nondominant side (usually the right hemisphere) only. The corticothalamic tract was carefully isolated so the surgery was not "blind." Only five of these patients showed little or no improvement, and eighteen made what the report called excellent postoperative adjustment. Some went back to work at fairly high-level jobs (one a high-level bank executive), and others functioned well outside the hospital. This was an older group of patients. No one accepted in the study could be under forty years of age nor older than seventy. Schizophrenics were also excluded since their (Washington University) experience with this procedure and chronic schizophrenia were mostly negative. One patient of the twenty-seven developed seizures (4 percent) controlled with anticonvulsant medications. Four of the twenty-seven showed some degree of cortical atrophy at surgery but still did well. Beyond the one patient who developed seizures, there was very little evidence of physical or mental impairment, and these were long-term (ten-year) follow-ups at an institution known for careful research.

Barohal (1958) reported on a five- to ten-year follow-up of 1,095 cases of prefrontal lobotomy done from 1947 to 1955 by the same surgeon on patients at the Pilgrim State Hospital in New York State. In those years, Pilgrim had a population of about fifteen thousand, many of whom were schizophrenic. The surgeon used the more careful "closed" approach (no ice picks) originally recommended by Freeman and Watts and similar to Moniz and Lima. There were 1,600 surgeries in that eight-year period, and 1,095 were available for follow-up from five to ten years. There was a control group of 606 patients recommended for lobotomy but from whom consents could not be obtained. At follow-up, 21 percent of the surgical patients and only 2 percent of the controls were able to live outside of the hospital. Those who remained in the hospital despite surgery were less violent and seemed to suffer less and had less trouble adjusting to the hospital. However, the rate of seizures on the operated group was 14 percent, either single events or multiple. Most were controlled by anticonvulsants, but Barohal felt they were directly related to scar tissue formation resulting from the surgeries. The death rate for the operated population was 6.2 percent related to the surgeries, which included a group for whom a cause of death could not be determined. Barohal felt these were "probably" cases of status epilepticus (prolonged seizure episodes).

At the time of the publication of this report in 1958, psychotropic medications had been introduced and lobotomies no longer done. Barohal's conclusions were that lobotomy would be a rare event in the future, but he could see that a few patients after failure of medications might be better off than otherwise. Barohal gives many case reports as part of this report. He gives rather detailed examples of longer-term adverse effects, which included weight gain (sometimes over one hundred pounds), disinhibition in sexual impulse and social expression, and memory loss for the period of the illness and sometimes before. Many patients did not show these personality changes and seemed clearly better off than before surgery. Several discussants at the end of this paper did agree that some patients seemed to benefit and were able to function outside of the hospital at relatively high levels. In the schizophrenic population, those diagnosed with "pseudo neurotic schizophrenia" did best. The question was whether the benefits overall outweighed the deficits overall. The conclusions were not easy to evaluate. Seizures and death were clearly risks. Death rates by suicide in schizophrenia and bipolar illnesses are in the 15 percent range and higher in some countries. I, personally, can only recall one patient whom I'd seen who had a lobotomy performed by Walter Freeman. The procedure was performed thirty years prior to my seeing her. It was difficult to assess if her impairment was a result of lobotomy or preexisting illness, but she had a lively personality and was no vegetable. Her record suggested that she had significant functional and behavioral impairments for years prior to her surgery, so there was no way I could conclude that, apart from a Babinski reflex (a sign of injury to motor neurons in the brain) on neuro exam, her problems were caused by her lobotomy.

Freeman (1957) published his own follow-up study. His was a report on three thousand patients followed between one and twenty years from 1936 to 1956. He compared patients in three different categories: prefrontal versus transorbital; private versus state hospital patients; and according to diagnosis: schizophrenia versus affective (mood) disorders versus psychoneuroses (anxiety disorders).

According to his report, the prefrontal approach resulted in 70 percent of schizophrenics, 80 percent of affectives, and 90 percent of psychoneurotics able to function outside of a hospital in the five- to ten-year period postsurgery. The rates were twice as high in private versus state hospital patients. He reported that the transorbital approach (his own technique) was safer (fewer medical complications) and less expensive and therefore better suited to state hospitals.

Ballantine, at Massachusetts General Hospital/Harvard Medical School Center for Stereotactic Neurosurgery in Boston, has published for years on his ongoing studies of over eight hundred cingulotomies (lesions made in the mostly anterior cingulate gyrus) for major depression. For most of my professional career going back forty years, Massachusetts General Hospital was the only site in the United States (to my knowledge) doing psychosurgery in any organized way, and I referred one patient to the program about twenty years ago. He suffered from intractable depression, had tried everything, and, having done his own research, asked if I would make the referral. I did. He did well for several years, relapsed, and went back another time before I learned about it. During the years that I followed him, he never developed any cognitive, neurologic, or personality changes.

In 1979, the National Commission for the Protection of Human Subjects of Biomedical and Behavioral Research reported on their review of over four hundred psychosurgery procedures done at Massachusetts General and found (Cosgrove and Rausch):

+ procedures efficacious in more than half of the four hundred cases
+ no psychological defects attached to these procedures
+ no evidence that minorities were targeted or procedures used for social control
+ in cingulotomies, pre- and postoperative studies showed improvement in full-scale, verbal, and performance IQ scores
+ detailed neuropsychological pre- and poststudies showed no deficits in all tests except somewhat lower scores on Wisconsin Card Sorting

In the 1950s, even as psychotropic drugs were being introduced and the call for these procedures was dropping dramatically, more accurate and precise techniques in stereotactic neurosurgery were being introduced. Brain imaging with the development of positron emission tomography (PET) and functional magnetic resonance imaging (fMRI) has become more sophisticated and becomes more so with each passing month. Lessons learned from the early years have been that the more focused and specific the symptoms targeted and the more accurate and minimal the lesions, the more minimal the side effects.

As of this writing and based on what the FDA is approving or overseeing, two disorders, which involve neurosurgical actions in the brain, are currently being investigated. One is severe and intractable obsessive-compulsive disorder (OCD), and the other is major depression, equally severe and intractable. This work goes forward because there are still too many patients seriously disabled by these disorders, and relatively specific "targets" have been identified. Schizophrenia remains the most complex and severe mental disorder, and a viable "target" in the brain has not been successfully identified other than those originally cited by Moniz.

In the case of OCD there is substantial literature going back over fifty years, using modern stereotactic techniques, which has reported some success with a specific area of the internal capsule (ventral portion of the anterior horn). Drs. Rasmussen and Greenberg at Brown University, and others around the world, have reported on the use of the Gamma Knife for OCD treatment, which is able to focus very small amounts of gamma radiation from multiple sources onto a single point (Aberlson, Curtis, and Saghar 2005; Kondziolka, Flickinger, and Hudak 2011; Taub, Lopes, and Fuentes 2009). The net result is ablation (destruction) of cells at the target but little harm to brain function as a whole (Taub, Lopes, and Fuentes). The Gamma Knife is used most commonly to target tumors in various organs in areas of the body that might be otherwise inoperable (e.g., metastatic lesions in the brain).

A newer technique, developed in the 1990s, that does not destroy brain tissue and is also reversible is deep brain stimulation (DBS). DBS has been used over the past twenty years, primarily in the surgical treatment of movement disorders like Parkinson's disease. It involves implanting a tiny electrode (or two electrodes if implanted bilaterally) at a very precise point

65

in the brain and applying a small electric current. The power source is, like a cardiac pacemaker, a battery implanted in the chest. If the procedure is ineffective, it can be removed.

DBS is being used in psychiatric research studies. Based on studies in brain imaging using PET and fMRI, researchers at Harvard and Cleveland Clinic have identified target areas for the treatment of OCD, which the FDA has approved for limited use (Reclaim system developed by Medtronics; Rauch, Dougherty, and Malone 2008; Greenberg, Gabriels, and Malone 2008).

The use of DBS for major depression, and more recently for bipolar depression, is also being explored through the work of neurologist Helen Mayberg, originally at the University of Toronto and now at Emory University in Atlanta, in collaboration with psychiatrist Paul Holtzheimer. Dr. Mayberg has earlier published research on the effects of antidepressant drugs on the functioning brain in real time using PET and fMRI (Mayberg 1997; Mayberg, Brannan, and Tekell 2000; Mayberg, Liot, and Brannan 1999). She identified specific areas in the brain that appear to change when patients respond to antidepressant drugs and when they don't respond. Her findings led her to collaborate with neurosurgeon Andres Lozano in doing DBS in patients with major depression. The patients who failed all available treatment to that point were selected by psychiatrists at the University of Toronto for the study. These were "unblinded" or open studies but seemed to show promise and with no evidence of personality change (Mayberg, Lozano, and Voon 2005; Lozano, Mayberg, and Giacobbe 2008).

When she moved to Emory University, a device company in Texas, Advanced Neuromodulation Systems (ANS, which in 2008 was acquired by Minneapolis-based St. Jude Medical), agreed to fund a multicenter study of DBS in major depression. Identified as the BROADEN study and approved by the FDA as a research protocol, the target is Brodmann area 25 in that part of the cingulate gyrus below the genus of the corpus callosum (for those readers unfamiliar with brain neuroanatomy, we'll just call it "deep" within the brain). This is different from the target used by Ballantine and Cassum at Harvard, although the cingulate gyrus is targeted in both. BROADEN is a double-blind research study at three sites, which later became fifteen sites. It began in 2008 with Helen Mayberg and Paul Holtzheimer as primary consultants. Alexian Brothers Behavioral Health Hospital was selected along with Columbia University in New York and

University of Texas, Southwestern Medical School, Dallas. As of this date, Alexian Brothers has implanted twenty patients. Our neurosurgeon is Dr. Konstantine Slavin, professor of neurosurgery at the University of Illinois, who is considered a "thought leader" by ANS and who performed the actual surgeries for the BROADEN study at Alexian Brothers Medical Center. All patients are followed for a total of five years.

Because of a very large anxiety disorder clinic at the Alexian Brothers Behavioral Health Hospital under the able direction or Dr. Patrick McGrath, we've become a major referral destination for patients with OCD. Dr. McGrath's area of expertise is anxiety disorders, especially OCD. Dr. McGrath is a psychologist whose training program at Alexian Brothers teaches techniques of exposure and response prevention to graduate students as well as patients. He sees some patients who are gravely disabled by their disorders despite competent and extensive behavioral treatment and medications for OCD, and who request that we do something more. In the past few years, we've had two DBS cases so far using the FDA-approved Reclaim system by Medtronics. Since 2006, a total of six patients have been treated using the Gamma Knife. So far only about 0.005 percent of this patient population might be considered candidates for either procedure, if that many.

Just as disillusion with science in the Romantic age did not stop the development of science in the nineteenth century, neither did the legitimate exploration of brain function in psychiatric illness completely stop the presumed excesses of the age of lobotomy, although it slowed dramatically. As you will see in chapter 10, American academic psychiatry in the forties and fifties did not see the brain (or human genetics) as having anything to teach us relevant to the practice of psychiatry, which added to the sense of outrage attached to doing anything with the brain. For the time, the brain was forbidden fruit, for both good and bad reasons. The views of a later psychiatrist/Nobel Prize winner are more in keeping with where psychiatry and psychiatrists are going today. Another twentieth-century development, psychotropic drugs (more forbidden fruit), will be discussed in chapters 8 and 14.

Frankenstein remains a metaphor today for various developments in the scientific frontier, not just in psychiatry. In the new areas of genetic modification we find Frankenstein corn, tomatoes, and other veggies, as well as human insulin (used safely daily by millions) created by Frankenstein bacteria (E. coli) of all things. Human-induced genetic modification, as

Darwin taught us, has been going on for millennia, taking the forms of collies, poodles, Siamese cats, and all manner of domesticated animals. And they have genetically modified some of us by virtue of the diseases they bring to us and how we've built resistance to them. We'll have to wait to see where it takes us, but we will most likely keep on looking. It is in the area of human genetics that psychiatry and neurology will most likely find the ultimate treatment for psychiatric and neurologic illnesses. It's important to remember that every cell in the body has the same complement of genes. Why, in the liver, do these genes create only liver cells and in the brain only neurons has to do with whatever it is within cells that activates some genes and suppresses others. Hopefully some latter-day Dr. Frankenstein will point the way without incurring the wrath of the gods.

It's important to understand that in the history of medicine it is rare indeed to do new procedures without problems, especially in surgery. Early mortality rates for gallbladder surgery exceeded 35 percent at the best centers in the late nineteenth century. Viennese surgeon Theodor Billroth, in the nineteenth century, did the first successful surgery for gastric cancer and gastric ulcers but not before many failures. Legend is that he was almost stoned to death in the streets of Vienna after the first patient he performed his Billroth I procedure on died. The Billroth I and II procedures are major surgeries with serious complications at every turn. Advances in medical (nonsurgical) treatment eventually reduced the need for that surgery, especially after the introduction of the H2 receptor blockers (e.g., Tagamet) and the more recent proton pump inhibitors (e.g., Protonix). Even before these newer medications, surgical techniques like vagotomy and pyloroplasty were supplanting the Billroth I and II techniques, which were horrendous surgeries and had major complications in the best hands. Where the Billroth still proves necessary, mortality secondary to hemorrhage and perforation still exceed 10 percent. In surgery these procedures are still done because there are no alternatives.

Siddhartha Mukherjee, in his 2011 book, Cancer:Emperor of all Maladies: A Biography of Cancer, chronicles the successes and failures in the last 130 years of attempts to understand and treat cancers of varying types. It took many years and literally billions of dollars before it became clear that many of the more radical surgeries for various cancers were of little or no value. But the genetics of cancer cells, like the genetics of mental illnesses, were not low-hanging fruit and are significantly more complex than the discovery of bacteria or the causes of malaria and yellow fever. If one compares the difficulty of finding cures for cancer versus mental illness, one would think that, after billions of dollars in research, cancer should be licked by now. With cancer one can actually look at cancer tissue and examine the morphology as well as actually map its very genome! How much more elegant can one get? And still each cancer is its own very unique process, so if we find a cure for cancer A, it may turn out to be of limited value in cancers B and C. Plenty of cancers are still not curable, but that does not diminish the value of treatment in prolonging life and contributing to the patient's quality of life where that is possible. The same concept applies to the treatment of chronic and persistent mental illnesses, except that for cancer, no one denies that its study is in the realm of science. For many years, up to and including very recently (as we shall see in a later chapter), mental conditions have been seen to belong more in metaphysics.

To try and fail is one thing. To not try, and fail, is quite another.

CHAPTER 7

A BRIEF HISTORY OF THE EVOLUTION OF HEALTH INSURANCE

From at least the time of Hippocrates and probably before, the relationship between doctor and patient has generally been understood as a strictly private one. However, as outlined in chapter 4, the longer training and adherence to the principles of science ultimately proved more expensive, eventually making the development of some form of health insurance inevitable. The Flexner Report, referred to earlier, dramatically reduced the number of operating medical schools in the country and developed high standards for those that preferred to remain open. The good news was that the quality of medical graduates significantly increased, and there was significantly less variance between the graduates of the best schools and the average schools. The worst schools went out of business when they couldn't meet the new educational standards. Higher standards in hospitals followed apace. The bad news was that there were fewer doctors, and high standards (in doctors and hospitals) came at higher prices. The Alexian Brothers' 58-cents-per-day costs are a distant memory.

Moreover, as surgical procedures became more heroic and as the expectations of better outcomes in nonsurgical illnesses requiring 24-hour nursing required more hospital time, the expense of hospitalization increased significantly.

Nevertheless, the concept of insuring the vast majority of Americans for hospital (and physician) care is relatively new. In 1900, the average American is estimated to have spent about five dollars a year for medical care, perhaps about one hundred dollars in today's economy (Umberg and Davison 2009). The real concern was lost income or business. Sickness insurance, such as that first issued by the Massachusetts Health Insurance Company of Boston in 1847, was primarily seen as coverage for lost wages since lost wages usually amounted to more than the treatment of the illness or injury (History of Health Insurance in the United States 2007).

In 1863, the Travelers Insurance Company of Hartford, Connecticut, offered accident insurance for railway travel, the precursor of similar policies offered today (History of Health Insurance Benefits 2002). In the 1870s, railroad, mining, and other heavy and dangerous industries began to provide company doctors funded by deductions from wages. The Mayo Clinic, for example, was situated along a rail line, which allowed injured railway and other workers access to treatment, especially in the case of injuries, which were many. As unions slowly grew in power and influence, workers gained access to company doctors or, as the International Ladies Garment Workers Union instituted in 1913, the country's first union medical service (History of Health Insurance Benefits).

Between 1915 and 1920, efforts to establish compulsory health insurance programs in sixteen states failed, but the real precursor of modern health insurance began in Texas.

In 1929, the Baylor University Hospital offered to insure 1,250 Dallas teachers at a cost of 50 cents per member per month, which would pay for up to twenty-one days per year of hospital care (History of Health Insurance in the United States). Strictly speaking, this was not health insurance so much as hospital insurance, which seemed to make sense since hospital care became more expensive (relative to physician charges) and could place one's economic survival at risk. As with everyone else in this country, for office visits, patients were on their own. This arrangement appeared to be win-win for all involved, so other hospitals soon followed suit. The Great Depression following the stock market crash of 1929 accelerated the need for hospital insurance since hospital costs did not follow the stock market.

In the 1930s, the nonprofit Blue Cross Blue Shield associations got started, essentially created by hospitals and doctors, and obviating the need for each individual hospital to set up a hospital plan à la Baylor University Hospital (Toland 2014; Scofea 1994). This gave patients more mobility and "outsourced" the insurance function. In the world of the 1930s, when most physicians were general practitioners and spent most of their time in the office or on house calls with relatively little time in hospitals, the idea of health insurance was viewed with suspicion and mistrust by most physicians. The idea of setting up large organizations to which would be given great quantities of cash and that would then promise to give some of it to the doctors ... well, physicians were generally a little paranoid anyway, and they just didn't feel right about placing a power source (money) in someone else's hands. When in 1935 medical insurance was proposed as part of the Social Security Act, physicians worked diligently to defeat it, and they succeeded until 1966, when Medicare was enacted. Prior to World War ll, however, few Americans had health insurance.

With the arrival of World War II, there was great competition among various industries for available workers (Scofea 1994). When the government instituted wage freezes, employers could compete for workers based only on better fringe benefits, and health insurance was one of those liked best by the workforce. With the rapid influx of workers in various heavy industries making steel and assorted instruments of war, new ways of paying for health care developed, and most of it was employer-based. Kaiser, on the West Coast, faced with the massive influx of workers in the absence of a large-enough established medical community, was quite creative and actually developed the first health maintenance organization (HMO). Kaiser, out of virtual necessity and for the first time, began explorations regarding what the term "medical necessity" might actually mean. The legacy of these times is that health insurance ever after became a function of employment, at least up to 1966.

The problem was that and individual or someone in that individual's immediate family had to have a job in order for them to have health insurance. Policies could be bought individually, as is possible today, though this is always very expensive because of the presumed risk pool of one individual. Insurance companies argued that only sick people would buy health insurance, and the healthy would see no reason for it, an argument that still finds traction today among the twenty-somethings. The term "moral hazard" is an insurance term, which means that the companies fear that consumers will buy insurance in order to afford treatment for a specific illness (e.g., having a gallbladder removed), after which the insurance is canceled. An analogy would be the restaurant owner who buys fire insurance as a prelude to setting fire to his restaurant. Generally, to have high-quality health insurance, someone had to either have a job working for a major company that could afford to buy insurance for its workers or work for a government agency since, as all public workers know (especially in Illinois), taxpayer resources are limitless.

Private sector unions were more powerful then and had many members, so labor negotiations at large companies paid particular attention to health benefits. Those who were self-employed or who worked for less affluent businesses generally didn't get wonderful benefits. But with more than half of the world's industrial production in 1946, it looked like the United States could handle it. Those who were too old to work, had no job, lost their job, or had children to support and no one to support them, well ... in Chicago there was Cook County Hospital; in Los Angeles there was Los Angeles County General Hospital, units one and two; and in New York, Boston, Milwaukee, New Orleans, and elsewhere, large publicly supported hospitals had been in existence for many years.

By this time in history there were many hospitals in cities of the world, and they were constructed in response to the perceived needs of the populations in those cities. The need was always there. The question was how was the community going to afford to care for those in need? When the Alexian Brothers built their first hospitals in Chicago and St. Louis in the middle and late nineteenth century, there was no health insurance, and two-thirds of patients were charity. The same was most likely the case at Presbyterian, Mount Sinai, Mercy, Swedish Covenant, Wesley, Passavant, and Provident. And if two-thirds of patients were charity, it was obviously the wealthier members of the German Catholic community who were going to fund this enterprise (Davidson 1990).

And fund it they did. Obviously the same thing happened in the Lutheran, Presbyterian, Jewish, Episcopal, Polish, Czech, Italian, Irish, and African American communities with varying degrees of success. The "haves" financing the "have-nots" has always been the case. The question wasn't if they were to be cared for but how well and how financed.

Writing of the period prior to 1941, Mayo Clinic historian Helen Clapesattle (1941) reports that, up to that time, 25 percent of all patients treated at the Mayo Clinic paid nothing at all. Thirty percent paid "the bare costs of their treatment," and 45 percent bore the cost for the whole. She goes on to say, "No note is taken, no mortgage is allowed, for the payment of a clinic bill, and no lawsuit is ever instituted to collect one." It was the Mayo brothers' opinion that every other doctor in the country did the same thing at that time in history and didn't see it as worthy of note. It is interesting that in the past twenty-plus years, among the most common causes of bankruptcies in the United States are medical bills.

With the growth of health insurance during and after World War ll, advanced medical care became more and more available to working Americans. Unlike some European countries, the United States did not "socialize" the practice of medicine. This was because we were relatively wealthy compared to most other countries, and we felt that, with health insurance spread liberally, we didn't need a government takeover of health care. In America, the solution was health insurance for those working and, in 1966, Medicare and Medicaid for those who weren't. The Medicare payment formula turned out to be unusually generous by today's standards. For hospitals it was "cost plus," which in effect meant that there was little incentive to control costs since costs (however they were calculated) were reimbursed plus a little more for "profit," which in a not-for-profit hospital is used for capital reinvestment and not dividends to stockholders. In the hospital industry these were known as "the good old days."

As an intern at the Los Angeles County General Hospital, unit one, in 1965/1966, I found the most notable change approaching the implementation of Medicare and Medicaid (Medi-Cal in California) to be a dramatic change in elective surgical cases as 1966 progressed. The repair of fractured hips (not exactly "elective" surgery) in the elderly had been one of the busiest services at Los Angeles County before Medicare and Medi-Cal were implemented. Later in 1966, it became one of the slowest. Clearly these procedures were now available at private facilities for what, before July 1966, was being done at county hospitals. From that point forward the great county hospitals would be in decline. Health insurance for psychiatric conditions was included in Medicare and Medicaid but with major restrictions, which will be more fully explored in a later chapter.

Another phenomenon presented itself at about this time. It was the for-profit hospital on a grand scale, as well as the for-profit health insurance company. Long a money-losing charity of sorts, the hospital was about to become a major profit center, highly desirable to an investment banking community not known for investment in charitable ventures. The 1960s and 1970s, as it turned out, became a time for serious moneymaking in the hospital world, even in psychiatry.

CHAPTER 8

PSYCHIATRY BECOMES LOCAL

When the Alexian Brothers came to Elk Grove Village, Illinois, in 1966, they used one of the wings in their new hospital for psychiatric patients, in keeping with their century's long tradition of working with psychiatric patients. Designated psychiatric units in general hospitals (St. Louis notwithstanding) were a relatively new yet growing trend in the United States at the time. Loretto Hospital on Chicago's far west side was one of the first hospitals in the United States to incorporate a psychiatric unit as a unique part of the original hospital design when built in the late 1930s. A few years after moving to Elk Grove Village, the Brothers bought a Four Seasons Nursing Home located across the street from the general hospital (called the Niehoff Pavilion) and converted the top floor into a psychiatric unit and the ground floor into a physical rehabilitation unit. An alcohol treatment unit (ATU) was also housed on a wing of the ground floor.

By the late 1960s, psychiatric units in general hospitals were not uncommon, made possible by shorter hospital stays associated with a few new psychotropic drugs, like the antipsychotic Thorazine, used in conjunction with antidepressants Elavil, Tofranil, and their derivatives. Another highly effective treatment for mood disorders, known as electroconvulsive therapy (ECT), was described in chapter 6. Treatments, which reduced the need for long periods in the hospital, lent credence to the hope that psychiatric disorders could be included in health insurance plans.

Between 1946 and 1974, the federal government was literally giving money away to local hospitals to upgrade their physical plants and build new facilities since a large portion of the population was moving to the suburbs. The legislation was known popularly as the Hill-Burton Act. This eventually resulted in an increase in hospital beds nationally and created some unused capacity at general hospitals. Some of that unused capacity was converted to psychiatric usage. Hospitals were happy to convert an unused wing to anything that might generate revenue, and companies formed that specialized in those conversions, as well as in the subsequent operation of these units.

Support for psychiatric coverage as a component of general medical/surgical health insurance was controversial from the start. The specter of a multiyear hospitalization, which was the norm for centuries and at older psychiatric hospitals considered of high quality, was an actuarial nightmare from an insurance perspective. The Kennedy administration and later the Johnson administration supported inclusion, though with specific limitations, which the medical/surgical components did not usually have.

The Community Mental Health Act of 1963 was also implemented by 1966, which had as its goal the treatment of the chronic mentally ill in the community (as opposed to the large state hospitals) through the funding of local community mental health centers (CMHCs). A movement toward treatment in the community, both inpatient and outpatient, for the bulk of psychiatric patients, public and private, seemed appropriate and promising.

A number of other developments in the medical treatment of psychiatric illness made their debut in the decades prior to 1966 and were discussed in chapter 6. However, the greatest impact began in 1954 with the introduction of drugs specific for use in psychiatric disorders.

The 1950s saw the development of the first psychotropic medications, referred to disparagingly as "chemical lobotomy" by some. It was a French pharmaceutical company (*Rhône-Poulenc*) in 1947 that synthesized the first phenothiazine (promazine) in the course of looking to develop a better antihistamine (Deniker 1970). From it, chlorpromazine was synthesized in 1950. It was first used by a French neurosurgeon, Henri Laborit, who described "sedation without narcosis," later referred to as "tranquilization." Laborit felt it was useful as an "anesthesia booster," but he saw in it some potential for use in psychiatric patients.

In November 1951, Laborit, in an ad hoc clinical trial of sorts, administered the drug to psychiatrist Cornelio Quarti, who described a positive tranquilizing effect. When he got up, however, he promptly fainted and felt the drug to be unsuitable for use in psychiatry. Laborit persisted, however, and in January 1952, it was used on a psychotic patient in a Paris psychiatric hospital who went from admission to discharge in just three weeks. The patient had dramatically improved. The problem was that this patient had also undergone treatment with ECT and several other drugs in use at the time, so the case wasn't exactly "clean" from a scientific perspective.

In 1952, French psychiatrists Pierre Deniker and Jean Delay published the results of a trial of chlorpromazine on thirty-eight psychotic patients using no other drugs or ECT and reported dramatic improvements on total doses of 75 to 100 mg daily administered intramuscularly. In 1953, Heinz Lehmann, in Montreal, reported on seventy psychotic patients treated in 1952 and 1953 with similar dramatic results for most. Deniker and Delay visited the United States, and in 1954, chlorpromazine began being used in American hospitals. The drug was approved by the FDA in 1955 for use only in postoperative nausea and vomiting. This is a good example, which occurs often, of a treatment that came into use well before the FDA officially gave its stamp of approval for use in another disorder. The positive effects of this early "off label" use initiated a revolution in psychiatric treatment that is still evolving, in that the next step was to try to understand why it was effective, which legitimized the renewed interest in psychiatric neuroscience.

This new drug had sedating properties with a very broad "therapeutic index." A broad therapeutic index is desirable, in that the dose required to sedate a patient is much lower than the dose likely to kill that same patient. In the fifties and earlier, various sedating drugs were used to treat agitated psychiatric patients whose therapeutic indexes were low. For example, if 100 mg of Pentothal, a barbiturate commonly used in psychiatry at the time, might sedate the average person, an agitated psychiatric patient might require many times that amount. The problem was that at 400 or 500 mg, respiratory depression was a palpable risk, and patients didn't always wake up.

The net result (with barbiturates and other sedatives) was that lower doses were routinely used, resulting in a greater-than-desirable frequency of the use of restraining systems such as wet towel packs, straitjackets, and five-point leather restraints. Also, lower doses of sedatives actually disinhibited patients (like alcohol intoxication) who then became even more out of control. Alternatives to the use of restraints were increases in patient/staff injuries. Psychiatric hospitals at times could resemble a pre-1846 operating room, but instead of minutes, this could go on for days or weeks or longer. Deaths from exhaustion during manic excitement did occur on occasion.

Enter the new antinausea drug chlorpromazine, which in the United States came to be known as Thorazine. This drug could sedate a normal person at 25 mg and an agitated psychiatric patient at 50 to 200 mg, and would be very unlikely to kill anyone at 2,000 mg, though the potential to lower blood pressure (as witnessed by Dr. Quarti, who passed out) made close observation important.

Safety alone made using this drug worth the effort. When it was discovered that the drug actually made a significant difference in the manifest symptoms of the psychiatric illness in just a few days, at least in its acute phase, the new age of effective psychopharmacology began. This development in some ways paralleled the development of sulfa or penicillin in terms of its effect on practice from that point forward. Here was a drug that seemed to target symptoms of the psychosis itself, beyond simply generalized sedation or tranquillization. This was different. Maybe there were discreet areas of the brain that could be targeted or influenced that could make a difference in these most elusive illnesses.

Suddenly after years of limited interest in psychiatry, major drug companies began looking at psychiatric drug development as a potentially profitable undertaking. Soon there were a multitude of chlorpromazine-like drugs being tested. One of these was imipramine (Tofranil). Its tricyclic molecular structure was very similar to chlorpromazine with seemingly only minor variation, but the drug turned out to be a disappointment in the treatment of psychosis. After being discarded as devoid of promise, Nathan Klein, at the New York State Psychiatric Institute, took another look and found the drug did indeed have minimal antipsychotic properties but reported rather noteworthy antidepressant effects (Healy 1998). Somehow the slight variations in the structures of these two molecules seemed to target the brain differently enough to influence two seemingly different conditions, leading to the investigation of "receptors" in the brain specific to drugs and neurotransmitters.

Another line of drug development occurred serendipitously while studying the effects of drugs used in the treatment of tuberculosis. In the early decades of the twentieth century, every city had its tuberculosis sanitarium, and large cities like Chicago and New York had many TB sanitaria. Like the old hospitals for cholera and yellow fever, these were as much for the protection of the well as for the treatment of the sick. True, rest and relaxation were part of the treatment of the disease itself (as in hundreds of other conditions), but the fact was that they were being quarantined from the healthy and often stayed there for years.

Naturally this separation from family, friends, and jobs, coupled with reduced income from not working, resulted in some very unhappy patients, and some became clinically depressed. When a new class of drugs came into use for the treatment of TB, someone noticed that the incidence of serious depression at these sanitaria seemed to go down. In addition to their action in the lung suppressing the tubercle bacillus (the TB bug), pharmacologic studies revealed that these drugs acted in the central nervous system by inhibiting the action of the brain enzyme monoamine oxidase. The net effect was to increase the availability and action of neurotransmitters like dopamine and norepinephrine in the brain. When these observations and published reports of the effectiveness of tricyclic and monoamine oxidase inhibiting drugs were eventually confirmed, the antidepressant drug industry was born.

ECT, the only truly effective biological treatment for depression and manic depression up to this point, was felt to be on its way out, along with the need for very long hospital stays. Psychiatric conditions seemed to be amenable to medical intervention in a more reasonable time frame, thereby making the treatment more cost-effective. The development of these new drugs (imperfect as they were and still are) affected psychiatry in ways reminiscent of antibiotics in medicine and sterile technique in surgery. The fact was that millions of sufferers of major psychiatric illnesses were able to lead more active and productive lives who might otherwise have been unable to do so, though it took time for these outcomes to be confirmed.

The relevance of these discoveries in the fifties and sixties meant that there was hope for community-oriented treatment in even the most severe forms of these illnesses. The argument that inclusion of psychiatric benefits in general medical benefits was unaffordable and unpredictable was becoming less tenable. Psychiatry was now becoming truly local.

CHAPTER 9

HEALTH INSURANCE, MORAL HAZARD, AND THE MARKET

In the 1980s, I served on the Health Insurance Committee of the Illinois Psychiatric Society. This was a committee developed in response to what was conceived of as an assault on the existence of insurance for psychiatric conditions by insurance companies and large employer groups. As part of this work, I, with other members of this committee, had opportunities to meet with representatives of several insurance companies and employer groups whose goals were to evaluate the place of psychiatric benefits in the overall health benefits market. Some of the views and opinions expressed in this chapter reflect these experiences.

As one can see from chapter 7, employer-based health insurance was a relatively recent development. There was no how-to manual, and the practical workability of the concept had not yet been fully explored. The original programs were first set up by hospitals, and later the "Blues" were not-for-profit organizations set up by hospitals and doctors to outsource the collection of premiums and payment of bills. One can easily believe that the original intent was a win-win strategy. The insurance function helped patients who became ill enough to require hospitalization afford the much more expensive care they needed and helped hospitals and doctors achieve more predictable financial stability. Unfortunately, insurance of any variety tends to make people much less concerned about cost.

Utilization guidelines in medicine and psychiatry were simply never thought of at that time in history. Surgical practice may have had a few restrictions, but generally there was little insurance interference. Tonsils and uteri (when women had the number of children they desired) were sometimes treated as bothersome and unwelcome and were removed upon request with questionable indications. The well-meaning but naive assumption was that all doctors who had similar modern training generally agreed regarding appropriate treatment. The prevailing view (by hospitals and physicians) came to be that the function of insurance was simply to pay for services and not evaluate whether or not they were necessary or effective. Except for those atypical or unusual health plans such as Kaiser Permanente in California (the earliest form of HMO), the role of insurance was to pay for whatever it was doctors and hospitals did and not ask too many questions. And at first they didn't.

Hospitals and doctors generally did not take the trouble to develop what are now referred to as utilization guidelines. What for? At this time in history, this was not considered the appropriate concern of health insurance. This was especially true in psychiatry, whose concepts and treatment techniques continued to baffle insurance companies, as well as our colleagues in the house of medicine. Definitions of psychiatric disorders seemed to most businesspeople (and many physicians) vague, arbitrary, and mysterious.

No matter. We knew what we meant.

Surgery, by contrast, was something of an exception, with tissue committees developing relatively early on. The goal of a tissue committee was to see to it that if an appendectomy or cholecystectomy (gallbladder removal) was performed, it was, in fact, the appendix or the gallbladder that was removed. They also acted as confirmation that they were, in fact, diseased, although in those days, before MRIs and ultrasounds, a good surgeon might expect a few "normal" appendices or gallbladders (though with gallbladders the surgeon couldn't always guarantee that removal of stones would necessarily result in relief of pain, which was why the surgery was being done in the first place). The uterus, however, could still be removed for "fibroids," which usually (yes, there were exceptions) caused no threats to life, liberty, or the pursuit of happiness. The same went for an anatomical condition referred to as "relaxed vaginal outflow" (RVO), which, as a student, I never quite understood (possibly a mild version of partial uterine prolapse). This unusual diagnosis I only encountered while moonlighting at a suburban community hospital doing presurgical histories and physicals. Few children during these years entered adolescence with tonsils or adenoids intact.

In general medicine, as in psychiatry, things were very often not so clear-cut either. Many diagnoses were referred to as "rule outs," and exact diagnoses, even after extensive investigation, were often never obtained, although the insurance form required something definite if one was to be paid for one's efforts.

Physician and hospital payment has always been very fluid, going back hundreds, perhaps thousands, of years. One couldn't just set some arbitrary price and expect to get it. Illness has never been a matter of election, and when ill, one needs treatment whether or not that person is capable of payment. There have always been practitioners who have had various "cures" and other treatments who could set their price and get it. This was generally not the case in a hospital setting, where one could expect to find the sicker patients with demonstrable pathology. Before health insurance the doctor or hospital did what it did and hoped to get paid whatever they thought the service was worth.

Hospitals in the Chicago area referred to earlier, set up by various religious groups, were set up to service a need, not to enrich their owners. They had to survive, however, and generate revenue, so they sent bills and tried to get paid. But it was clearly understood that not all, maybe not even most, would be able to pay. Before health insurance, physicians took care not to use the hospital arbitrarily since cost has always been an issue. Moreover, a costly hospitalization might also leave the patient with less to pay the physician, and physicians have never felt an obligation to enrich hospitals. Call it a kind of enlightened self-interest.

Health insurance eventually brought the concept of "medical necessity" into the lexicon. Without a third-party payer, why bother with the term? If the doctor recommended it, and the patient wanted to go ahead with it, whose business was it but these two? One could question the effectiveness of the treatment: Is purging an effective treatment for heart failure? Operating for centuries under a humoral theory of disease (expelling one humor [i.e., fluid or secretion] to rebalance another), perhaps one could make a case for it. Scientific advances in the eighteenth, nineteenth, and twentieth centuries questioned the effectiveness of many time-honored treatments, but "medical necessity"? Why would the patient see the physician if there was no "medical necessity"? That just didn't compute.

Once health insurance is in place, one can then ask if the hysterectomy for relaxed vaginal outflow, or not wanting any more children, is medically necessary. The question is now appropriate if we're going to ask an insurance trust, union, or self-insured company to spend the risk pool's resources to get it done. Will the prospect of a stockpile of money waiting to get spent make hospitals, doctors, or patients more likely to undertake procedures for convenience (hysterectomy) or curiosity (MRIs, CT scans), or because the patient wants antibiotics or wants to avoid lawsuits (every conceivable lab and imaging study). This is what insurance companies refer to as "moral hazard." Another example of moral hazard is the patient who gets a job to accomplish something like gallbladder surgery, only to quit the job after the surgery and recovery have been accomplished. One doubts that this was very common, but it did exist, and the result, to protect the insurer, was the practice of not insuring preexisting illnesses or of having long waiting periods before a preexisting illness would be covered, if ever.

Before the recent changes mandated by law in the Affordable Care Act (Obamacare), it was impossible for some patients to ever get health insurance. The need for health insurance made it impossible for some patients to change jobs or otherwise advance in their profession for fear of being uninsurable because of a preexisting condition. Whatever controversy engendered by this legislation, it appears to allow sick people (i.e., those who actually need it and whom all insurance companies try to exclude) to get health coverage.

The insurance companies of course have had some moral hazards of their own (e.g., profit margins and stock value) to contend with, like trying to enroll healthy populations and avoid potentially sick ones since the for-profit insurance company owes its primary obligation to its stockholders and not to its enrollees. In fact, its abiding obligation now and forever will be to avoid "losses" (insurance jargon) and maximize profit, which means that sick patients are best avoided by whatever means. Insurance companies have never seen this as a moral hazard, but of course it is. If a patient becomes ill and goes to a hospital, there is no alternative to treating him. If a person needs health insurance but cannot afford it, no insurance company sees it as their obligation to insure a nonpaying patient. The very thought of it is deemed absurd.

Payment for physician services became based on the concept of "usual and customary," which in day-to-day practice meant that the doctor who charged more got paid more and those who charged less got paid less, regardless of their skills and experience. This was, in my opinion, a well-intentioned effort by insurers like Blue Cross to allow patients free choice access to presumed experts (i.e., "specialists"), as well as a recognition of the "market" in that, in the absence of insurance, it might be that physicians in places like New York or Washington or Chicago might command higher fees than practitioners in rural areas, for example. Therefore, if one lived in a more affluent area but was not affluent, one's choice of physician did not have to be based on price. Who wants the cheapest surgeon? The very question seems inappropriate when it's your abdomen (or chest or brain) being cut into even though there turns out to be actually very little relationship between price and quality when looking for a physician (or hospital, for that matter).

The net result, however, was that it was impossible to tell which physicians were better than those who were "average." Doctors who'd just finished training and were least experienced but needed to establish a "usual and customary" charged the most, and those with the most experience tended to charge relatively less over time—basically the opposite of most other professions or trades.

For hospitals, many of which had been established before the arrival of health insurance, it was whatever the traffic could bear. But, as a rule, without health insurance the traffic couldn't bear very much. Costs were always an issue. Many years ago my mother worked at a local hospital operated by Catholic nuns who in those days took care to control costs by having as many unpaid nuns as possible do as much of the routine work as possible. That was possible in times when nuns (and brothers) were plentiful, relatively uneducated, and willing to devote themselves to a life of manual labor and service as an expression of Christian charity. There are far fewer nuns (or brothers) today who are much better educated than they were then. Now, of those who are left, many are well-educated hospital administrators (although still probably not paid much beyond what's required in order to be eligible for Medicare when they retire) who generally no longer work in the laundry (usually outsourced) or kitchen (seldom outsourced but often managed by outside organizations).

With the advent of private health insurance and (what turned out to be) a generous Medicare and private insurance payment strategy, the hospital went from expensive charity to profitable enterprise if one considered location, population served, and services offered. Stock offerings lured investors with the prospect of excellent return on investment. For-profit hospitals claimed that "increased efficiencies" and superior management would justify their place in the marketplace, essentially claiming that super profits would come from the money saved by these presumed efficiencies.

Another issue related to the concept of moral hazard is what I refer to as "ethical stewardship." This term refers to the appreciation on the part of physicians, hospitals, and patients of the fact that Ford, General Motors, Motorola, the states, and the federal government have created large pools of cash (insurance or tax monies or self-funded trusts) to be used for the benefit of employees, the sick elderly, the disabled, or the poor. Ethical stewardship refers to an awareness that professionals have an ethical duty to understand that these well-intentioned resources are not infinite and represent someone's (or something's) hard work, tax payments, and goodwill. There should also have been the awareness that those who give can also take away if costs get out of control, and the perception develops that the best interests of the patients are being subordinated to the best financial interests of the providers.

In time and with costs inevitably increasing above that of inflation generally, doubts began to arise about the value payers of medical services were getting for dollars spent. As a medical student in the early sixties rotating on a clinical service, one felt one could always tell the interns (as they were called then) from the residents by the length of the orders written on new admissions. If the interns wrote ten, the residents wrote twenty. If the intern was good for twenty, then no self-respecting resident could do with less than forty, which seemed to be a demonstration of superior knowledge. Cost just didn't seem to be an issue. The more obscure and numerous the rule-out diagnoses, the smarter the doctor, or so it seemed. Although this was common practice at publicly funded city and county hospitals, in private settings (in the good old days) insurances paid for each test individually.

As a medical student working my way through school, I and other medical students earned money by moonlighting at local community hospitals, doing histories and physicals on presurgical patients. It seemed that, at community hospitals, everyone got what they wanted. By day at the medical school, students were taught to have a legitimate, evidenced-based reason for every medical or surgical intervention. How surprising, it turned out, to see that some women were having hysterectomies for what amounted to anxiety, depression, birth control, or simply personal preference. For patients whose symptoms didn't respond to the usual remedies in the family doctor's office, it was common practice for a patient to be admitted on Sunday night and examined by the primary care doctor on Monday morning. A host of tests and consultants would be ordered: neurology for headaches, gastroenterology for tummy pain, ENT for nasal symptoms, orthopedics for back or joint pain, cardiology for chest issues, and so on. If nothing was found, a psychiatrist possibly would be called for an "urgent" consultation on Thursday or Friday. The "urgency" was the patient's expectation of discharge by Friday. Many hospitals were full Sunday night to Friday and relatively empty from Friday night to Sunday night, like hotels, when they began to fill up again.

The glory here was that everyone was happy! The patients were happy for all the attention, even if little was found (although someone always found something). They loved their doctor for being so "thorough." The consultants loved the primary care doctor for calling them in on the case. The hospital loved the doctors for not only bringing the patient to the hospital but ordering all those individually billed tests and x-rays, in more recent times maybe an endoscopy suite, or in the best of all possible worlds an operating room. Incentives were clearly perverse. The circumspect doctor who took care to only do what was necessary might be disparaged by the patients for lack of thoroughness or for simply not agreeing to give the patient all that he or she wanted. The thoughtful doctor struggled, while the other prospered. There was no incentive to use resources wisely, as the patient's and the doctor's sense of entitlement increased over time. The reaction by the paying community when it inevitably came in the mid-1980s was called "managed care."

CHAPTER 10

THE ASCENDANCY OF PSYCHOANALYSIS IN AMERICAN PSYCHIATRY

We must recollect that all of our provisional ideas in psychology
will presumably one day be based on an organic substructure.
—Sigmund Freud, On Narcissism (1914)

The deficiencies in our description would probably vanish if we
were already in a position to replace the psychological terms
with physiological or chemical ones. We may expect [physiology
and chemistry] to give the most surprising information and we
cannot guess what answers it will return in a few dozen years
of questions we have put to it. They may be of a kind that will
blow away the whole of our artificial structure of hypothesis.
—Sigmund Freud, Beyond the Pleasure Principle (1920)

As mentioned in chapters 8 and 9, health insurance for psychiatric conditions has always been controversial. The reality in psychiatry has always been long stays, often years in an asylum or "sanitarium" and, as such, had been the case for centuries. Medicine in the nineteenth and early twentieth centuries made major and very palpable advances based on careful observation and description, coupled with sometimes elegant, inductive reasoning. In the absence of diagnostic imaging and a modern high-tech laboratory, observation and description were critical and efforts often rewarded with major discoveries. Careful laboratory studies of the nervous systems of animals and humans were relatively highly developed by the 1890s.

Even in nonsurgical and nonpublic health medical practice, hormones were discovered and isolated, germ theory was refined, the role of vitamins in health and illness was detailed, and in the 1930s and 1940s antibiotics were developed, known as "miracle drugs" in my childhood. In the nineteenth century, pathological examination of organ tissue, grossly and microscopically, showed the workings of diseases in various organs of the body, even if little could be done.

Study of the brain demonstrated the effects on behavior of brain infections, tumors, war injuries (especially during and after World War I), and impaired blood flow. These were significant discoveries gained by disciplined thinking and careful study. In psychiatry these brain discoveries came to be known as "organic" symptoms, the area where psychiatry and neurology overlapped. Regardless of symptom presentation, if pathophysiology could be identified, it became a neurologic disorder. If no pathophysiology could be identified, it became a psychiatric or "functional" disorder. In the functional psychiatric conditions (in most organic neurologic conditions, as well), therapeutic discoveries were slow and often disappointing. In neurology one could often demonstrate a "lesion" or map out a specific area of sensory or motor dysfunction. However, cognitive/emotional dysfunctions were something else again.

The central nervous system in general seemed especially resistant to major breakthrough in terms of effective treatment. The specialty of neurology went through a kind of golden age in the later nineteenth century as the neurologic exam was refined and, as all medical students witnessed, was taught with a certain haughtiness by professors of neurology because of its (relatively) exacting precision. Motor and sensory lesions could be more or less precisely located by careful neurologic examination, even before MRIs, x-rays, and other imaging studies were available. However, what one could actually do about many of these afflictions was very limited, and while localizing a disorder may be professionally satisfying, curing it was another matter. The other problem is that the brain has more than just motor and sensory areas.

Many neurologic disorders are degenerative in nature, and the list of truly treatable neurologic conditions by 1900 was not a long one. A "curable" list essentially did not exist, though some just got better on their own. Surgery again was something of an exception, in that some disorders, like abscesses, tumors, and traumatic injuries, were accessible neurosurgically with varying degrees of treatability and occasional cures.

Even by 1965, beyond epilepsy, movement disorders, and ADHD (treated primarily by neurologists in the 1950s and 1960s), the treatable list was very short and the list of untreatable conditions very long. Bacterial infections could be cured with the advent of antibiotics, and the treatable list is longer now but (neurosurgical interventions excepted) not much longer. Stroke is a good example of a condition completely untreatable when I graduated from medical school (1965), but it has become very treatable if treated promptly today. My younger sister died recently of a rare neurologic disorder called cerebro-basilar degeneration. It was progressive, debilitating, and ultimately excruciatingly painful for her physically and almost as painful for her family to watch. The lesions were bilateral (both sides of the brain), more or less localizable on neurologic exam, and visible on MRI. But there was simply nothing that anyone could do about them. The brain is extraordinarily complex and not easily influenced. The "easy" discoveries have been made. The low-hanging fruit has been picked.

In the nineteenth century, the distinction between neurologist and psychiatrist was blurred. Sigmund Freud, a neurologist and neuropathologist, trained in Vienna in the 1870s and 1880s, hoped for an academic career at the University of Vienna. He studied at Ernst Brucke's Physiologic Institute, where he did research, gave lectures, and wrote papers on nerve cells. Brucke had several young assistants already and advised Freud to consider actually practicing neurology if he ever hoped to marry and be able to afford a family.

Starting as a resident at the University of Vienna Hospital in 1883, he met the eminent brain anatomist and professor of psychiatry, Theodor Meynert, who was impressed by Freud and asked him to work in his Laboratory of Cerebral Anatomy (Sulloway 1979). Freud accepted and worked there from 1883 to 1886. During these years, he published a paper on cerebral hemorrhage and the medicinal uses of cocaine, including its worth as a topical anesthetic (Freud 1974; Sulloway).[10] Freud found the study of neuroanatomy more precise and exacting than psychiatry, which he found "unfruitful" and unstimulating after a five-month stint in Meynert's psychiatric clinic. Sometime later he also became an expert in and published papers on the paralytic disorders of children (Freud 1968).

Freud applied for and won a fellowship to study neurology with the French neurologist Jean-Martin Charcot in Paris (October 1885 through February 1886), the "Mecca of Neurology." On Tuesdays and Fridays, Charcot gave lectures on nervous diseases at the *Salpêtrière*, a Paris psychiatric hospital where Freud learned about the use of hypnosis in so-called "hysteria" patients. Charcot believed that all psychiatric disorders, including hysteria, had their origins in forms of brain dysfunction, even if not yet discovered. Through hypnosis Charcot could remove symptoms, add new symptoms, and then remove them again. Charcot knew that these patients were not cured by these demonstrations.

These lectures and demonstrations prompted Freud's interest in what he later referred to as the "unconscious." Freud was so impressed by Charcot that he named his oldest son after him. Charcot showed great interest in the psychopathology (psychiatric aspects) of diseases and, by his fame, legitimized its study in neurology.

Upon returning to Vienna, Freud began to collaborate with the highly accomplished former neurophysiologist and now–general practitioner Josef Breuer, who also seemed particularly interested in patients suffering from hysteria. Breuer was clearly the senior partner in this collaboration. His work in the laboratory of Ewald Hering resulted in Breuer's discovery of the role of the vagus nerve in respiration, now referred to as the Hering–Breuer reflex. Working with physicist Ernst Mach, Breuer discovered the critical role in balance of the fluid of the three semicircular canals of the inner ear.

---

[10] Freud's work on cocaine turned out to be a problem for him in that he didn't seem to recognize its potential for abuse. He used it himself (as did Sherlock Holmes/Conan Doyle) and apparently never became addicted, but others were not so fortunate. One was a friend who was addicted to morphine whom Freud attempted to treat using cocaine. Freud came under some professional criticism for this, having traded one addiction for another. Freud's discovery of cocaine's potential as a topical anesthetic for surgery led to its being pursued and developed for eye surgery by a friend Carl Koller. Koller eventually claimed full credit, so, in cocaine research, Freud lost out in both areas.

Breuer's patient, known in the psychiatric literature as Anna O., was of particular interest to Freud and stimulated him to study patients of his own with similar symptoms of hysteria.

Medicine in the 1890s was not as specialized as it is now, but patients tended to be referred to those with neurological training because of the manifest impairments in sensory and motor functioning. Hypnosis was a commonly used technique by Freud, Breuer, and others, and there was general acceptance of the notion that sexual problems were a common etiologic agent in symptom generation. This was not a Freudian discovery.

Together, Freud and Breuer published Studies on Hysteria in 1895. Their developing differences about whether sexual issues usually (Breuer) or always (Freud) were causative in hysteria eventually caused them to part ways. It was also the case that Breuer was a busy general practitioner and couldn't devote the considerable time required to seeing such patients. Freud developed the theory that inappropriate contact between his patients and opposite-sexed parents was the cause of symptom formation in cases of hysteria. This is called "trauma theory" in psychoanalytic history. He initially believed that this was an important discovery.

Between Studies on Hysteria in 1895 (and earlier) and the publication of his book The Interpretation of Dreams in 1900, Freud developed the foundations of psychoanalysis. At first his views of mental functioning were right out of the physiology lab. Nervous energies "built up" and demanded "discharge." When that couldn't happen for some reason, the mind "displaced" these excitations into somatic symptom formation. Since these processes were "unconscious" (a term Freud got from Breuer), symptom removal required that they become conscious so that the conflicts that made these thoughts or memories unacceptable are made less unacceptable. Psychoanalysis at this stage saw mental conflicts in a kind of "economic" model (I have preferred the term "hydraulic"), with pressures in one part of the system resulting in actions or "displacements" in another. Freud tried very hard during the years prior to 1900 to understand the operations of the human mind in biological terms. He asked appropriate questions: Why sex? How were these experiences repressed (made unconscious)? How was choice of neurosis determined? His attempts to find answers to these questions resulted in the development of psychoanalysis.

It is generally agreed that 1900 is the year of the official birth of psychoanalysis. Over the next forty years, psychoanalysis became more complex as Freud moved away from a physiologic model, which he and later followers found too limiting, to a more "dynamic" psychological model. Freud was not well accepted in European academic medical circles, although he was widely read in the nonmedical world.

Freud felt that psychoanalysis had little to offer those suffering from the major psychoses, today known as schizophrenia, bipolar illness, and severe major depression. But as referenced by Sulloway (1979), Freud had written several papers trying to include paranoia and the hallucinatory psychoses as examples of rather extraordinary "defense mechanisms" in psychoneuroses. He also wrote his interpretation of a book written by one Herr Schreber, who clearly had a paranoid psychosis (Freud 2002). Freud did not say or imply that psychoanalysis could do anything for these patients. But since Freud apparently saw the same defense mechanisms in operation in serious psychoses, some later analysts adopted the notion that diagnosis in psychiatry, unlike every other disease or disorder known, was irrelevant, and only the method of treatment was of any real importance.

In phenomena as mundane as the act of forgetting and slips of the tongue, Freud saw evidence of the workings of an unconscious mind. The point here is that in the unconscious there are no accidents. Its advocates saw psychoanalysis as central to a comprehensive theory of mind rather than merely a way of understanding mental afflictions. As such, its importance went beyond mere medical application.

Freud, the consulting neurologist, understood that the emotional life was housed in the brain and that all psychological phenomena derived from its workings. Despite the progress, the neuroscience of the time was inadequate to explain how the brain went about creating "mind." There was too little understanding of how the emotional brain worked and offered psychoanalysis as the best method for explaining what we could observe, i.e., the thoughts and behavior of the patient's sometimes tortured, but relatively coherent mind. Moreover, as a neurologist, he saw the kinds of patients who came to neurologists in his time, who were very likely to be different from those seen to populate the psychiatric facilities of the day.

In The Interpretation of Dreams (Freud 1900), he proposes that in the dreams of the relatively normal are the experiences of what, in the waking state, might be considered psychotic. However, the primary interest of the book is not psychosis, in which he was not particularly interested, but rather his interpretation of how the unconscious affected dreams and everyday waking life. It was, in effect, a study of normal mental (mind) processes. Freud was one of those rare prolific geniuses who, despite only publishing (after 1900) on six or seven case histories, was able to write twenty-two volumes of psychological/psychoanalytic work, which mated a theory of causation to a method of treatment to a method of training for the treatment. Psychoanalysis was nothing if not comprehensive.

Freud became influential worldwide for the same reasons as Charles Darwin. Darwin's name is associated in the popular mind with "the theory of evolution," whereas, in fact, Darwin's contribution was to elucidate the method by which evolution is purported to occur (i.e., "natural selection"). There were many publications advocating the idea of evolution before Darwin was even born (one by his paternal grandfather, Erasmus Darwin) and many before Darwin ever published on the subject. He distinguished himself by methodically presenting evidence for his views, and in much the same way so did Freud. At least in the beginning, he didn't start out with a theory that he was determined to prove but rather developed his theories based very closely on what his patients presented. As a "hard" scientist he was trained to follow the evidence, and that's clearly what he attempted to do.

Freud was greatly influenced by Charles Darwin's evolutionary thinking, as was virtually everyone in the world of biology and medicine. Freud personally owned Darwin's Origin of Species (1859), The Descent of Man (1871), and The Expression of Emotions in Man and Animals (1872), and according to Sulloway (1979), they were well annotated, and Freud made no secret of Darwin's influence. The fact that Darwin could demonstrate the similarities in emotion and in emotional expression between "lower" and "higher" beings on the phylogenetic hierarchy supported the notion that these early developmental "drives" and instincts were hardwired even in humans and served some survival/reproductive purpose. There could also be consequences if they were interfered with or damaged, pointing the way to the relevance of studying child development and its deviations. In the Darwinian view there are only two tasks of any consequence in biology—survival and reproduction—and the more intricate and elaborate of these two from the perspective of the emotional life is the latter.

In my view, the problem with psychoanalysis was that Freud wasn't

Darwinian enough. To understand my meaning here, one has to understand that Darwinism and evolution are not one and the same. In fact, the evolutionary theories of Jean-Baptiste Lamarck (1744–1829) remained highly influential despite Darwin, especially because Darwin did not have a viable theory of genetics up to the time of his death in 1882. The debate about whether or not evolution had, in fact, occurred was an issue only for the religiously pious. For the academic community the issue was not so much whether, but how, it occurred. Lamarck's theories had been around for many years and seemed to explain the evidence.

Lamarck's view was that the internal physiologic "needs" of an organism and its efforts to satisfy those needs drove the process of evolutionary change. For example, the giraffe lived in an environment where pasture became less available for long periods of time, and it had a "need" to eat foliage that was available only in trees. Its efforts to eat forced it to make efforts to stretch the herd's collective necks, which became an acquired characteristic of giraffes that each generation passed on to the next, each generation having a longer neck than previous generations. This was much quicker than the method proposed by Darwin by many eons and seemed to make sense. By the same thinking, if a man (or woman) lifts weights rigorously and grows large muscles, his/her offspring would be more likely to have large muscles. Lamarckian evolution implied movement toward long-term "improvement" of species. In other words, evolution always went "forward." To Freud, "necessity" became the power of unconscious ideas over the living systems (humans and otherwise) and implied an "omnipotence of thought," which actually could result in a psychoanalytic explanation of evolution. Wow!

Even Darwin was forced to accept some degree of Lamarckian influence in evolution in later editions of The Origin to satisfy his many critics. The answer to his critics lay in the pages of an obscure German science journal in the 1860s, written by a Catholic monk of all people, that apparently no one ever read or understood. By 1900, the genetics that Darwin needed to prove his theories were developed independently, and Gregor Mendel's experiments with peas were finally acknowledged. Lamarck was on his way out and with it the power of psychoanalysis as a factor in evolution.

Well, not quite. Freud liked Lamarck well into the twentieth century. Modern genetics is rather esoteric and not very sexy. In 1958 (or thereabouts), I saw a TV program purporting to show, through "evolutionary theory," what humans would look like in one hundred years (2058). By that year, humans are predicted to have even larger heads but much smaller bodies. Increased brain use would "necessitate" larger brains, and the absence of a need for physical labor via robots, TV remotes, and universal car ownership would result in a shrinking muscle mass (and the complete atrophy of our fifth toes). Watson and Crick? Double helix? DNA? Maybe not. Viva Lamarck!

Meanwhile, and as popular acceptance grew, psychoanalysis appeared to offer insights into the major social and political movements of the time (as did something called social Darwinism) and could be espoused, opposed, or at least commented upon by Marxists, Socialists, Liberals, anarchists, and others looking to remodel society in a new paradigm. Many came to believe that psychoanalysis was sufficient to explain virtually every human mental activity not merely in psychiatry and psychology, but in philosophy, art, literature, religion, politics, law, economics, and foreign relations, to name but a few.

Freud's theories gave infantile sexuality a central place in the diagnosis and treatment of psychoneurotic disorders. He didn't do this because he was a dirty old man or some kind of pervert. He came to this conclusion because this was where the evidence seemed to point. Like other physicians of his time, he believed that human sexuality began around puberty. When the evidence seemed to point in a different direction, he acknowledged his mistake and moved in a different direction. He came up with his particular version of infantile sexuality, which was not in and of itself an idea original to Freud.

Nevertheless, these ideas were controversial and met with some resistance, as one might imagine. His supporters argued that his assertions about childhood sexuality was the reason his writings met such resistance in Vienna (Catholic and conservative), Berlin (Protestant and conservative), and elsewhere in Europe in medical and nonmedical circles. This, Sulloway (1979) writes, was not true. His Interpretation of Dreams was actually very well received in nonmedical circles. In the medical community, where someone is always proposing some new idea, there is always resistance to new ideas (as seen with Dr. Semmelweis in chapter 4) until the mechanisms are explained and debated and the results confirmed repeatedly by others. In medicine, this is business as usual and always will be.

But there was also the problem of the strength of the evidence and whether or not the available evidence could withstand critical debate and lend support to conclusions being made. In the professional community, exposed to all manner of unusual theories and ideas about illness at that time in history, psychoanalysis, as a therapeutic undertaking, could be legitimately criticized on scientific grounds.

Briefly, psychoanalysis in its original form was based on Freud's observations that under hypnosis he was able to resurrect certain thoughts and memories that the patient did not seem to be aware of when fully conscious. It further seemed probable that these "unconscious" thoughts and beliefs had considerable influence in the waking life and behavior of the patient. Up to this point these observations were not original to Freud, having been made by writers as varied as Friedrich Nietzsche and William Shakespeare, as well as other neurologists working with patients whose symptoms appeared to have no anatomic (based on what was known about the brain at the time) basis.

Freud went beyond hypnosis and felt he'd discovered, through what he called "free association," a method superior to hypnosis in getting at the unconscious thoughts, fears, and beliefs of patients he treated. Through this new method he believed he was able to posit the developmental stages of early human emotional development and argued that certain traumatic influences at the various developmental stages, if not sufficiently resolved, would manifest themselves as "neurotic" symptoms in subsequent years. Patients would report on their dreams and other notions and thoughts revealed during these periods of free association while awake. Freud asked his patients to say whatever came to their mind during their sessions with him, no matter how whimsical or silly they might seem. He saw this technique as ultimately superior to hypnosis.

In the Interpretation of Dreams (Freud,1900), he saw dreams as a manifestation of the unconscious mind unfettered by the demands of consciousness. The book was methodical and detailed and, like any good work of medical science, examined the scientific literature on dreams up to that time and explored all possible sources of error that he could think of. It received enough attention at the time to assure his place as one of the great thinkers of the period, and it remains a monumental work of original thinking to this day.

However, as with any other new scientific idea, it required replication and confirmation. It did offer a new way of looking at common problems that presented in the offices of neurologists and other physicians, and still does. Soon others were at work trying to reproduce and verify his findings, which depended heavily on how the putative analyst interpreted and responded to whatever was produced by the patient. These were not laboratory-based, well-controlled, scientific undertakings supported by large research grants, which in any area of clinical medicine was uncommon in that age. On the contrary, the process of replication and confirmation was quite informal and involved attempts on the part of various physicians, neurologists, psychiatrists, and so on to try the procedures and report results at meetings or publish the results in journals. Many journals came into existence during this era serving various medical specialties, including psychoanalysis. This was not unlike the manner in which most areas in medicine or surgery were rapidly and dramatically advancing.

Science historian Frank Sulloway, in his 1979 book Freud, Biologist of the Mind, gives us a fascinating look into the medico-scientific trends of the late nineteenth to early twentieth century. Sulloway presents evidence that, instead of being shocked by his assertions about sexuality, some in the medical community thought Freud's ideas to be reactionary rather than revolutionary. They thought they had gone beyond blaming disorders on sexual impulses, and Freud seemed to be reasserting what they regarded as no better than the resurrecting of old superstitions. But there was more to Freudian theory than the resurrecting of old superstitions.

Controlled experiments in clinical medicine, especially at that time, were difficult or impossible to perform. The usual method was careful and thorough observation and description, by which such methods had produced major discoveries. In areas like pathology, it was fairly straightforward: examine a diseased organ or tissue grossly and then microscopically. Correlate the symptoms of the patient with the diseased organ or tissue in gross and microscopic terms, maybe backed up with photographs of the patient and then the tissue. Someone read the article or listened to the lecture and found another patient with the disease, examined the tissue, and reported on his results. And so it went. If subsequent results were as originally reported, there was agreement and eventual consensus. If the results were different, there was controversy. Maybe the original report was wrong. Maybe the patient's diagnosis was incorrect. Maybe there are variations of that particular disease previously unreported. Just another day in the world of medicine: describe, discuss, compare, reexamine, replicate, verify, and develop consensus.

In psychoanalysis, the process was the same but the method difficult to standardize or replicate. Given the potential for variation in observation and interpretation, it became necessary to try to standardize the observer. Hence, the analyst needed to be trained to make the salient observations. This came to involve a personal analysis, preferably by Dr. Freud himself or someone trained by him. His followers saw things in their patients that they felt Dr. Freud missed (Jung felt that memories of early sexuality were created by patients after puberty and presented as if from childhood), so there were variation and disagreement over what the "core" features were and ultimately a lack of consensus.

The time needed for analytic treatment initially wasn't excessive. But as time went by, the analysis began taking longer and longer as new issues and problems were identified and as it became apparent that "superficial" analysis was not having the once-hoped-for curative effects. Whereas Joseph Lister was able to report a reduction in mortality from about 50 percent to about 15 percent, as a result of the adoption of sterile surgical technique, the goals and hoped-for outcomes in psychoanalytic treatment were often difficult to pinpoint. Admittedly, reporting on who died and who did not is rather straightforward and lends itself to neat data collection in surgical conditions. However, it would have been nice to develop some more precise definitions of success and failure in terms of conditions and methods. Maybe that couldn't happen at the time, but it probably explains at least in part why psychoanalysis was not impressive to Freud's medical colleagues, sexual content notwithstanding.

The actual treatment process in early Freudian psychoanalysis involved two important and essential components:

- analysis of the patients' natural "resistance" to the process of freely associating and laying bare all things, no matter how upsetting, and accepting analytic interpretations
- analysis of the "transference" (i.e., the tendency in all patients to eventually form a conception of the analyst based on their own previous experiences and "trauma" of childhood); development of a so-called "transference neurosis" was deemed essential to any

successful treatment, and it was said that cure was not related to an intellectual understanding of oneself and past trauma, but more to an emotional "working through" (another term difficult to define), as it were, of these primitive experiences in the light of analytic understanding

Symptom formation depended upon the complementary roles of fixation and regression, which were clearly psychological concepts but based in biological research, some of which was done by Freud himself on brain damage in children (Sulloway). He reported on three forms of cerebral lesions: traumatic (physical, traumatic injury to the brain, usually by accidents), vascular (via circulatory disturbances), and inflammatory (infections). Outcomes in all three forms he felt to be "inhibitions in development" of surrounding brain tissue (fixation) or regression to earlier levels of development.

Freud's view on regression came via the English neurologist John Hughlings Jackson (1835–1911), who had a strong evolutionary view of nervous system development. Jackson saw the mind-in-brain as a hierarchical structure with "higher" voluntary functions maintaining continuous control over "lower" involuntary ones (Sulloway). This was an evolutionary development ultimately leading to the primacy of humans in the animal world. In mental illness, dementia, and various neurologic conditions, there occurs a reversal in this process with a regression to earlier developmental levels. These regressions are seen normally on a temporary basis in sleep and in dreaming.

The postulated phases of early child development in Freudian psychology were oral, anal, and phallic/Oedipal. The cognitive correlates (how the child understands and mentally processes) of the events in one's life may not necessarily correlate with real circumstances and may be greatly misinterpreted. Nevertheless, that is how the infantile mind works. According to theory, these early childhood experiences can form the bases of later neurotic distortions in adulthood if experienced as traumatic.

An example of rather benign pre-Oedipal thinking in childhood is the following: Many years ago I was supervising a resident at Loyola. He related a story about an experience with his child, who was about three years of age at the time. It was the time of the Watergate hearings, and Richard Nixon was still the president. Father and son were both in front of the TV one night, and father was watching the hearings, which were the riveting news events of the day. The son was playing on the floor, seemingly interested in why his father was so engrossed in the TV. According to his father, the boy then suddenly became very focused on the TV and began shouting, "Nixon did it! Nixon did it!" When his father responded, "What did Nixon do?" the boy said solemnly, "He went pee pee in his pants."

The presumably controversial part of Freudian theory was his conception of the sexual content of the Oedipal stage of development, in which he believed that children in this phase had sexual fantasies about their opposite-sexed parents (or possibly parent substitutes). Freud initially believed that the parents (or parent substitutes) of his patients actually had inappropriate sexual contact in some way with these patients in childhood. This is referred to in analytic history as the "seduction theory." The reactions of patients, he thought, resembled a post-traumatic reaction brought on by the awakenings of sexuality at puberty. Freud felt very uncomfortable with this delayed-reaction theory and felt it didn't explain enough to make the data credible.

If this did happen, why did it not continue? Why the fantasies around this period only? Certainly these things could have happened, and no doubt have happened more than we'd like to admit. But could this be the major cause of neuroses? Were the boys abused by their mothers, as well? Neuroses (a term not used professionally these days, having gone the way of "lunatic") do occur in males.

Freud finally came to decide that the fantasies were real but the behavior was, by and large, not. This was new. If these fantasies are universal and not simply manifestations of post-traumatic stress, then what we have here is what he labeled an "Oedipus complex," and sexuality is somehow hardwired (due to some evolutionary necessity?) in the brain and manifested earlier than anyone had expected, perhaps even into earliest infancy. So why do girls have fantasies about being rescued and loved forever by handsome princes, and why do boys enjoy fantasies about rescuing damsels being besieged by dragons and other assorted monsters? Is it possible to make peace with a dragon? In Freud's view of a properly "resolved" Oedipal stage, yes. If not properly resolved, it would be no, and we are then doomed to keep creating dragons into adulthood. Are these observations just cultural peculiarities related to the ways in which we teach children to respond to fairy tales and gender roles and are unrelated to biological development? Current evidence simply does not support a biology-neutral view, in my opinion.

In more recent decades, some feminists have taken to blaming Freud for his abandonment of seduction theory, as if Freud was somehow personally responsible for the last hundred years of father/daughter (and mother/son?) sexual abuse by labeling the victims as neurotic. The Oprah Winfrey "school of pop psychology" has been especially vocal in popularizing these new outrages.

If some of psychoanalysis's basic theories might be considered at least possible, they were difficult to prove definitively in the manner of Pasteur's work on the growth of organisms or Walter Reed's work on malaria and yellow fever. Unlike what was happening in surgery and public health at the time, there were no data to support the cure rates of one analytic technique over another. Given the eventual plethora of theories, it sometimes seemed as if "cure" was irrelevant so long as one's theory seemed vindicated. Today, very few patients are in classical psychoanalysis, but theories of psychotherapy and the origin of emotional disorders abound. There is little doubt (in my mind) that psychoanalysis was helpful to many patients. It is also true that other techniques and theoretical approaches have also been helpful.

The European scientific community basically thought it was interesting work but much of it not testable or falsifiable and hence, by definition, unscientific. One had to believe it to study it, which made it look more like a religious, philosophical, or political movement than science. And what, in the end, did psychoanalysis tell us about major psychiatric disorders like schizophrenia or manic depression or severe major depression? It didn't provide any more than one could have learned some other way. The potential margin of error was just too much for mainstream scientific acceptance.

In general medicine too there was not universal agreement on what constituted illness and health. In the waning years of the nineteenth century, there were various fads and movements, founded on questionable scientific investigations, which saw the development of different directions in health care. It was at this time in history that varieties of "cures" were espoused by advocates of various stripes, which gave rise to schools like chiropractic, naprapathy, homeopathy, vegetarianism, and various "movements" that either have not survived or survive as "alternative treatments" with a very flimsy evidence base. The introductory lecture at the University of Illinois in September 1963, which began my junior year in medical school, was given by Dr. Max Samter, an internist who was a popular teacher and a major contributor to the medical literature of the time. He cautioned students who were about to begin their clinical years that the Oracle of Delphi in ancient Greece reported a 90-plus percent cure rate. Twenty-three centuries later, despite significant progress in scientific medicine, we were most unlikely to come anywhere close.

But, while Freudian notions were received lukewarmly in the capitals of Europe, they were very positively received in the United States. It's difficult to say why, apart from the fact that we know that unconscious motivations influence us. There are various reasons given for American psychiatry becoming so taken with psychoanalysis, while most European academic communities were not. In 1909, Freud was invited to America to give a series of five lectures at Clark University, which were very well received. Freud, sorry to say, was not impressed, and he never came back. Freud unfortunately thought of America as an intellectually barren place populated by legions of the newly rich who were inclined to chase the latest European fads, liked to conduct séances, and were easily impressed by humbug. Freud, apparently, was not immune to snobbery.

Nevertheless, interest in psychoanalysis grew steadily, and, between roughly 1940 and the 1970s, psychoanalysis became the dominating influence in American academic medical schools, when career advancement and professional standing depended on psychoanalytic training (Kandel 1998). The "best" training programs in psychiatry were psychoanalytic in orientation and the best teachers' analysts, or so it was believed. The study of neuroscience was no longer seen as premature (Freud's position) but simply irrelevant (Kandel 2006).

So why did psychoanalytic thinking become so popular in the United States? One thought (I can't recall the reference) was that America was different from Europe in that it became a destination country for millions of European immigrants from about 1830 to the 1920s, when immigration was severely curtailed. These immigrants, after about 1880, were perceived by many to be subverting the very fabric of the American way of life as it was being conceived and were viewed as a significant threat by those whose ancestors had come to America only a few years earlier. The new (1880 to 1920) arrivals were largely Eastern and Southern Europeans. Social theories of the time took on a kind of social Darwinian character coupled with some bizarre, but sometimes fervently believed, theories about race, ethnicity, and genetics. Notions of a need to control the reproduction of the "unfit" were popular and became known as the "science of eugenics." The more they came, the more reactionary ideas began to take hold.

These theories were more likely to be debated in America than in Europe since America was on the receiving end of these migrations. Being a nation founded on principles of "equality," many found it difficult to accept traditional notions of static social position or cast, and at the same time they were not especially happy about the influx of millions of foreigners. Certainly these new arrivals presented cultural challenges. They were Catholic, Orthodox, or Jewish; spoke different languages; and sometimes brought over European revolutionary ideas like Anarchism and Marxism, which traditional Americans viewed with suspicion and alarm.

Psychoanalytic thought became attractive to those who wished to challenge these pseudoscientific and reactionary ideas regarding race and ethnicity, because psychoanalysis implied that we were more alike than different and our personalities and ideologies a result of early learning and child-rearing rather than biology (breeding). While the French Revolution and the plethora of subsequent (usually failed) revolutions in many European countries by 1848 showed that traditional ideas of class and privilege were clearly under attack, they were still more likely to be openly challenged and/or debated here in America, in response to these reactionary social and biological intellectual movements. Maybe the "melting pot" needed an intellectual counterforce to social Darwinism.

Enter here also various other intellectual and social movements of the late nineteenth and early twentieth centuries. The importance of culture, learning, child-rearing, education, and other influences was recognized and better appreciated than it had been before. Behind it was the notion that in America, regardless of the circumstances of one's birth, the possibilities were unlimited. The result for psychiatry was that it became more and more identified with social and political causes and less identified with scientific medicine, especially after World War ll. The appearance of psychoanalytic advocacy of the primacy of early learning and experience, seen through an expanded and reinterpreted psychoanalytic microscope, came to explain everything to some psychiatrists, social theorists, sociologists, and psychologists.

Psychiatry as a medical specialty merged with and attempted to explain the various social and political movements of the time and often became identified with them. While psychoanalysis certainly did not give rise to the revolutionary movements, it did purport to give insight into their origins. Writings such as Freud's Civilization and Its Discontents (1961), The Future of an Illusion (1961), and Moses and Monotheism (1961) quickly became part and fabric of the political and intellectual debates of the time.[11]

In the absence of better science, psychoanalysis in all its permutations became attractive and was no doubt enhanced in prestige by virtue of its presumed medical (i.e., scientific) origins. In a world where the pathophysiology of disease after disease was being understood, and incredible progress was being made on many fronts, psychoanalysis appeared to say something profound about the issues of the day and appeared more intellectually challenging than in the static world of traditional psychiatry, where hopelessness seemed endemic.

Even psychiatrists with strong interests in brain research had an interest in and/or felt their careers required psychoanalytic training. Eric Kandel, Nobel Prize winner in physiology and medicine in 2000 for his pioneering basic research on memory, is an example of a psychiatrist who found himself interested in psychoanalysis. In fact, his only reason for going to medical school at all was to become an analyst (Kandel 2006). When he first went to Harvard, it was to major in modern European history and literature. He met a girl, Anna Kris, whose parents were both psychoanalysts (Ernst Kris and Marianne Kris) and were educated in Vienna. Marianne was a close friend of Freud's daughter Anna, after whom her own daughter was named. Through the Krises, he met some of the most renowned names in

---

[11] Even outside the psychoanalytic world per se, as in newly Bolshevic Russia, psychiatry became politicized as a way of saving dissidents from Stalin's executioners. In the 1920s and 1930s, soviet psychiatrists were certifying that those who openly criticized Comrade Stalin and the dictatorship of the proletariat were not traitors but merely madmen who needed psychiatric therapy to be helped to understand the error of their ways. Unfortunately, that ploy ultimately backfired when the Communists, having lost millions of citizens before (Stalin's terror) and during World War ll (an estimated 28 million casualties) moved away from executing dissidents, instead placing them in mental hospitals for "treatment."

psychoanalysis and found these discussions fascinating and exciting. For the study of mind, it was the only game in town except maybe cognitive psychology, which seemed less dynamic and exciting.

However, his biological studies in medical school forced him to begin looking at the biology of the brain, and he got hooked. He says he went into basis science research because he found it fascinating and because he felt that even a psychoanalyst should know what's going on in the brain. Kandel felt that even abstractions like ego, id, and superego represented different cerebral operations (as did Freud), which could one day be understood. For Kandel, Freud's observations represented possibly the best of nineteenth- and early-twentieth-century observational medicine that could and would someday be translated into modern neuroscience. He was surprised by how little interest most analysts showed in the operations of the brain. By this time in history, psychoanalysis was a purely psychological enterprise, and all Darwinian or genetic influences were deemed irrelevant.

Kandel's is an interesting odyssey from undergraduate in European history and literature, to medical school, to psychoanalysis, to neuroscience and a Nobel Prize.

With the biological "revolution" occasioned by the development of effective psychotropic drugs after Thorazine came a widening rift (always present to some extent) between "psychoanalytically informed" psychiatrists and those who were not so "informed," with patients often caught in the cross fire. Even within the Freudian camp itself there were those who argued that Freud's ideas were essentially biological and those who argued that biology had no role in things psychiatric. These were fervently believed.

While the development of effective psychotropic drugs brought with it the prospect of being able to treat fairly serious psychiatric conditions locally and reduce hospital stays from sometimes years to months or weeks, the influence of psychoanalysis was such that essentially two varieties of psychiatrist came into being, even before the widespread availability of health insurance:

- Those who used predominantly a medical model of treatment and tended to use somatic treatment were more likely to be found in state or private hospital practice. Like their colleagues in general medicine, where specific causes of many diseases were unknown, tended to treat patients symptomatically and were thought of as "superficial" or "failed Freudians" as the fashionable magazines of the time sometimes referred to them. This group felt genetics in psychiatry had an important role to play, as did biological research.

+ Those who espoused a psychoanalytic or psychotherapy model and were to be found primarily in office practice (though with some very famous hospital affiliations). They saw themselves as treating the "root causes" of symptoms with what they liked to refer to as in-depth dynamic psychotherapy. The implication here was that we could know the specific (psychological) causes of psychiatric disorders if we only had the proper training and knew how to read the telltale signs. This group felt genetics had little, if any, role to play in psychiatric conditions, and physiologic research was basically irrelevant and a waste of time.

With the panoply of psychiatric conditions presenting for treatment at any given moment, each group tended to find patients who would seem to reinforce their particular model. Both groups believed fervently in their models. In my opinion, health insurance or financial gain had little to do with the issue, at least not at this time in history, since those in training were taught their particular models with the best of intentions.

Nevertheless, in choosing places to train in the 1950s and 1960s, one was essentially choosing a point of view based on one's understanding of psychiatry and what kind of knowledge it had to impart to students.

Medical students' points of view were, to a large extent, affected by where one went to medical school. The "best" programs at that time, with some notable exceptions, were believed to be psychoanalytic in orientation, or so the students at the University of Illinois believed, since that was the information available. Psychiatry was seen by many as a branch of knowledge that was primarily concerned with the study of "human nature," with only an occasional glance at conditions like schizophrenia or manic depression, which the majority of faculty avoided since such patients made very poor psychotherapy candidates.

Since the intellectual foundation of psychoanalysis was based on a developmental model of human emotional development (oral, anal, and phallic/Oedipal stages of development), and since the manic-depressive symptom picture was difficult to fit into a developmental framework and still make sense, manic depression (now called bipolar illness) simply ceased to exist in many university settings. Schizophrenia could fit into the analytic developmental model (schizophrenia was the most "primitive" form of mental illness and its fixation point earliest [oral stage] in development), so there was a good deal more schizophrenia diagnosed than manic depression.

At the University of Illinois in the academic year July 1, 1966, to June 30, 1967, of about one hundred patients (in total) admitted to the inpatient services, only one carried a diagnosis of manic depression. An interesting topic of discussion among residents of the time was why there were so many more manic depressives in Europe (and everywhere else in the world) than in America. The notion was simply that, as in all other areas, we were simply ahead of the rest of the world. In 1970, the introduction of lithium in the United States brought an astoundingly rapid change in the incidence of diagnosed manic depression.

Eric Kandel reviewed the situation. In his 1998 article titled "A New Intellectual Framework for Psychiatry," Kandel writes that after World War II, medicine was transformed from a practicing art into a scientific discipline based on molecular biology, while psychiatry went from a medical discipline to a practicing therapeutic art. Academic psychiatry, Kandel writes, "abandoned its roots in biology and experimental medicine and evolved into a psychoanalytically and socially oriented discipline that was surprisingly unconcerned with the brain as an organ of mental activity."

It depended on one's point of view. Psychoanalysis believed it taught psychiatrists respect for the patient's thoughts, feelings, and personal/social history. The patient as a person, not just a disease (diagnosis often irrelevant), was good for patient and doctor alike. It no doubt led to considerable creativity and attracted some very brilliant students who explored new ways of looking at human functioning, in those with mental illnesses and those without.

Its approach could be called "humanistic," in the tradition of the Italian Renaissance humanists, if not in the tradition of Lister, Broca, and Virchow. Moreover, there is little doubt that some patients are treatable only through psychotherapy; and for some, most "medical" treatments are inappropriate. For many more patients some form of psychotherapy is always appropriate in addition to medical treatment. Even with the major psychoses, psychotherapy can serve a function similar to physical rehabilitation after stroke or other physical injury. As we'll discuss later, there is developing evidence that psychotherapy can positively influence brain function in its own right. But whether or not specific psychoanalytic insights were relevant was still an unsettled issue. Nevertheless, the insights that psychoanalysis seemed to give into human mental functioning seemed more exciting and interesting than what was available using a medical model.

However, while being humane and compassionate and intellectually stimulated is a good thing and makes a good therapist, it doesn't necessarily help in understanding mental illness as a medical condition, which most serious forms clearly are. Many a physician has stood at the bedsides of dying patients in centuries past who would have preferred to offer something more effective than compassion alone if given the choice.

In the same article cited above, Kandel reports on his experience as a beginning psychiatry resident at Harvard's esteemed Massachusetts Mental Health Center in 1960. He had just come from postdoctoral work in neural science at the National Institutes of Health. He described his training at Harvard's Massachusetts Mental Health as "leisurely" with no required or recommended readings. "We were assigned no textbooks, rarely was there a reference to scientific papers in conferences or in case supervision. Even Freud's papers were not recommended reading for residents ... Reading, they argued, interfered with a resident's ability to listen to patients and therefore biased his or her perceptions of the patients' life histories." One often-quoted remark was "There are those who care about people and there are those who care about research." Guess who the good doctors were?

Kandel goes on to say that there were no grand rounds at Massachusetts Mental Health and no outside speakers invited to address the house officers on any regular basis. It was not until 1965 that grand rounds were initiated at Massachusetts Mental Health (at the insistence of the residents), and when they requested a speaker on the genetics of mental illness, they could not find a single psychiatrist in all of Boston who was concerned or ever seriously thought about the subject. "We finally imposed on Ernst Mayr, the great Harvard biologist and a friend of Franz Kallmann, a founder of psychiatric genetics, to come and talk to us." Psychiatry as a branch of medical science was all but dead at Harvard in the early 1960s. But the residents were ahead of the faculty, and Kandel maintained his interest in neuroscience. Along the way he developed five principles, which he believes will prove to enhance our understanding of the biological bases of mental processes:

1. All mental processes are neural.
2. Genes and their protein products determine neural connections.
3. Experience alters gene expression.
4. Learning changes neural connections.
5. Psychotherapy changes gene expression.

Given his background, it is impossible to believe that Dr. Freud would have taken issue with any of these points, at least prior to 1920. Nonetheless, in most academic departments of psychiatry in the era where psychoanalytic thinking was preeminent, the use of any biological treatment was often seen as, at best, "superficial" and perhaps unworthy of the prestige of the institution. At worst, it could be seen as patient assault and a possible manifestation of negative "countertransference" on the part of the doctor who only did these things to patients he didn't like or looked down upon as unworthy of psychotherapy. Some other very famous training centers in the United States, such as the Menninger Clinic in Topeka, Kansas, moved away from a medical model of illness in favor of a psychoanalytically based system. The result was, in 1963, Karl Menninger's book, The Vital Balance, which argued that all psychiatric classification should be abolished since in mental illness, "perhaps there is only one class of mental illness-namely, mental illness" (Kandel 2006). In effect, no matter what the condition, the treatment was the same: psychoanalysis with certain modifications.

Freud himself, however, argued for the usefulness of psychoanalysis in some severe cases of major depression and manic-depressive illness. In his 1917 publication Mourning and Melancholia, he explores the relationship between normal mental processes (grief) and abnormal ones (melancholia):

> The most remarkable peculiarity of melancholia ... is the tendency it displays to turn into mania accompanied by a completely opposite symptomatology. Not every melancholia has this fate ... one would be tempted to exclude these cases from those of psychogenic origin, if the psychoanalytic method had not succeeded in effecting

an explanation and therapeutic improvement of several cases of the kind. It is not merely permissible, therefore, but incumbent upon us to extend the analytic explanation of melancholia to mania.

Freud's standard of proof becomes "several cases" that improved.

Psychoanalyst Dr. Thomas Szasz took the demedicalization thinking of the time to its most obvious and logical (nonmedical) conclusion, when in 1961 he published what he became most famous for, a book titled The Myth of Mental Illness. The book's title was its premise: there is no such thing as mental illness in the way we were using the concept of medical illness. The only proper concern of physicians is "real" disease, which is always associated with material changes in the brain and the body. Szasz concluded that since proper pathophysiology had not been identified, we were unlikely to discover what probably did not exist. Therefore, terms like "schizophrenia" were merely labels invented to justify incarceration and control of those who chose to be different. He seemed to be saying that if we didn't understand the medical/molecular/genetic basis of schizophrenia by 1961, then it was unlikely that we ever would. In the absence of good neuroscience, it became one opinion versus another—a debate among medieval scholastic monks or rabbis about how many angels could exist on the head of a pin.

Szasz was particularly upset by the use of the diagnosis of schizophrenia, which he felt was invented as a pretext that allowed the state to incarcerate and "treat" persons against their will when their ideas differed from the majority of the population. He argued against the concept of syndrome-based diagnostics in psychiatry even though it was common practice in most other areas of medicine. He proposed that the "lesion" was the hallmark of disease in medicine, the absence of which in psychiatry made psychiatric diagnosis an absurdity. He was somehow able to ignore the fact that most diseases began as syndromes and became full-fledged diseases when definitive pathophysiology was finally identified. There was no such thing as hypertension before the invention of the sphygmomanometer (blood pressure cuff), although there were symptoms and sequellae, which were subjectively experienced in various organ systems before we were able to divine cause and effect. Pain is another example of a symptom with varying etiologies and expressions, some of which are known and many of which are not. Was malaria a myth for thousands of years before we learned that the "cause" had to do with mosquitoes?

Szasz advocated the abolition of laws regarding involuntary hospitalization and argued that every choice by every individual on the planet was a free choice that should be adjudicated in the same way all the time. There should be no insanity defense, because insanity is, after all, a metaphor. The person either committed a crime (e.g., Oedipus) or didn't, and that should be the only issue before the court. Suicide is a free choice and should not be interfered with. So was the use of heroin (Szasz avoided the issue of allowing fourteen-year-olds free choice of heroin and suicide).

Psychosis was a form of "malingering" by which a person sought to gain attention from those around him. He compared the notion of involuntary hospitalization to the historical persecution of Jews and homosexuals. He claimed that the Nazis would prevent Jews from committing suicide only to save them for the gas chambers. These Jews and homosexuals may have chosen suicide as a preferable alternative to Nazi work camps and associated humiliations. Since suicide may have been a rational choice under these circumstances, does that make every suicide a rational "free choice" in every case?

Szasz died in 2012 at the age of ninety-one. He managed to ignore the overwhelming scientific evidence of genetic and other biological influences in schizophrenia. If the concordance rate of schizophrenia in identical twins is 50 percent and in fraternal twins 15 percent, there is obviously some kind of genetic influence operating here that goes beyond how one is raised. He raised many important issues, however, about how we treat mental patients, and many of his concepts eventually became incorporated into mental health law. It was the apogee of the mind versus brain dualism, which has had such strong influence in psychiatry for the last one hundred years. Dr. Szasz apparently never heard of Charles Darwin and evolutionary science. Apparently every organ and component of every living thing on Earth went through biological/evolutionary influences except the human brain, which functions not in the realm of biology but of metaphysics.

In one of those bizarre twists of fate, Szasz's insurance company in 1994 paid out $650,000 to the widow of one of his patients who had a known bipolar illness and was on lithium (Kandel 2006). The patient had allegedly been advised by Dr. Szasz to discontinue lithium, after which the patient hanged himself with battery cables. By 1994, it seemed that juries were not buying the "free choice" theory of psychiatric illness any longer. Lithium has since been shown to be psychiatry's most effective antisuicide drug.

By the time I became a resident at the University of Illinois in 1966, things had changed somewhat, and the "better" programs had come to understand that some of these newer treatments had scientific merit, and residents had to be taught to use them, however reluctantly. The chair of psychiatry was Melvin Sabshin, who was a psychoanalyst (everyone was) but also a real educator for whom psychoanalysis was not necessarily revealed religion. Dr. Sabshin invited junior and senior students interested in psychiatry to his office on a monthly basis to discuss what was going on in the field and allowed a critique of what his staff was saying in lectures and clinical psychiatry rotations. No axes to grind; no oxen to be gored. He was a true educator and, in my opinion, an erudite gentleman who later became medical director of the American Psychiatric Association. As such, he became the face of American psychiatry in government and in the profession worldwide for the next thirty years.

At this time in history (the early 1960s), programs with a psychoanalytic slant saw no influence of genetics in any form of "functional" mental illness, and for medical students the only lectures on psychotropic drugs came as part of pharmacology classes given in the sophomore year only. Our predominantly psychoanalyst faculty could teach us nothing about psychotropic drugs (nor did they wish to), though we read what was available in pharmacology textbooks. However, the overall education in general medicine and pharmacology was so good that it was not difficult to learn what we needed to know. Our final exam in psychiatry was mostly about "mechanisms of defense" (presumed cause of all psychiatric symptom formation) and psychoanalytic theory and nothing about anything having to do with the brain or the new psychotropic drugs. They clearly didn't matter.

In 1966, with the weight of evidence beginning to tilt in the direction of at least some value to biological treatment, the university felt it had to teach residents about the rational use of the new drugs. As it happened, a recent graduate of the psychiatry program at Washington University (St. Louis), Dr. Robert Leider, came to Chicago to begin classes at the Chicago Psychoanalytic Institute. Washington University in those days was considered a maverick institution, in that they unashamedly espoused a medical model of psychiatric illness. Dr. Leider obviously felt he needed more training on the other side of the spectrum.

While I realize that the simile is flawed, I'm going to argue that psychoanalysis was a bit like the Catholic church in 1500, and Washington University was like Martin Luther. The flaw is that the Catholic church in 1500 represented traditional Christianity, and in the 1950s and 1960s, Washington University to a great extent represented traditional medicine. Psychoanalysis was considered the reform movement.

The faculty at Washington University espoused "hard-core" research in genetics and psychopharmacology, long-term follow-up to determine the natural history of psychiatric syndromes, and little need to tailor psychiatric research to the needs of (in their opinion) philosophical and political theories. Our faculty saw Washington University as an inferior program, but if they knew nothing else, they knew about drugs, and Dr. Leider's job was to teach us what we needed to know.

Electroconvulsive therapy had not been used at the University of Illinois in the memory of any of the existing faculty. There was a rumor that someone in neurology had used it a time or two in the past, but no one could say for sure, since we never spoke to neurologists, who were rumored to inhabit the north tower of the university's two-tower Neuropsychiatric Institute. Psychiatry inhabited the south tower, and although the architecture of the building, as well as the name (Neuropsychiatric Institute), implied collaboration with neurology, we never saw one of them, not even for a consultation. As it happened, members of the famous Gibbs family, creators of voluminous and widely read EEG atlases, were still in the building (basement). Several residents went on "safari" one day and actually found them!

The average length of stay for psychiatric patients (at the University of Illinois) in those years was about nine months (we felt it was too short), some longer and a few shorter. In the residency class just before 1966, some patients stayed for three years, or the entire residency-training period of a resident. Cost was not an issue. Neither was service to the community. The issue was superior training of residents, and it was felt that the taxpayers of Illinois were best served by turning out superlative doctors who would ultimately treat relatively few patients but treat them very well.

The average first-year resident saw perhaps eighteen, maybe twenty, patients max the entire year. Like Eric Kandel's experience at Harvard's Massachusetts Mental Health Center, the pace was "leisurely." Although we had many classes, we were encouraged to read classical analytic papers, and there was excellent psychotherapy supervision that, in every case, was the treatment. Drugs were used to make the more psychotic patients "amenable to psychotherapy." Psychotherapy, as practiced here, was not meant to be merely supportive in the sense we use that term today. The goal was something called "insight," though we understood that "cure" was only possible in a true psychoanalysis, which was beyond the expertise of residents and the capacity of the more seriously ill patients we saw as inpatients.

The senior faculty were exclusively office-based, but very infrequently we were asked to hospitalize one of their patients who would be seen in the hospital by a resident. One patient had been seeing a senior attending five days per week for about ten or more years. This particular patient was fairly high functioning and held a position as comptroller of a medium-sized Chicago corporation. The senior attending left whatever medication the resident thought might be necessary to the discretion of the resident since the very act of prescribing was thought to be a confounding element in the treatment and best left to someone else. This patient's treatment had reportedly been the origin of a number of papers written by the attending psychiatrist as contributions to the analytic literature.

When the residents reviewed this case as part of a "grand rounds" and questioned the frequency and long years in analysis, the attending felt confident in asserting that, without the analysis, the patient would undoubtedly have been inhabiting the back ward of some state hospital and be completely nonfunctional. We were asked to accept this assertion as a matter of faith (the revealed religion component in psychoanalysis) since there were absolutely no longitudinal studies that could be cited to support notions such as these.

The better hospitals of the period were (in no particular order and leaving out many): McLain, outside of Boston; Sheppard-Pratt, Baltimore; the Menninger Clinic, in Topeka; Chestnut Lodge, outside of Washington, DC; and in Chicago, Michael Reese P&PI, where Roy Grinker Sr. had been chief of psychiatry. He had been analyzed by Sigmund Freud himself. What characterized these "best" of all institutions were long stays, often amounting to years, and a strong belief in psychoanalytic theory as the centerpiece of therapeutic intervention. There were calls for psychiatry to throw off its "medical mask."

The prestige of psychoanalytic treatment during these years was such that it became common (some might say fashionable) for writers and other artists, since time immemorial seen as particularly "neurotic" as a corollary of their creativity, to pursue psychoanalytic therapy. Woody Allen would become something of a caricature of the artist-in-analysis, but it was very common. Whether analysis enhanced creativity or suppressed it is still a matter of debate, but creativity was seen to originate in the unconscious, and the analyst held the franchise to that part of the mind just as securely as the surgeon to an open abdomen.

To those in the creativity business, appearance is sometimes more important than substance. In the art world, how creatively the answer is pursued is often more important than whether or not the answer is, in fact, correct. This, of course, is antithetical to the goals of scientific inquiry. In analysis the patient is encouraged to free-associate, and whatever comes out of that process, once analyzed, is seen as truth of a sort. No matter that there can be myriad interpretations of these data, each can be true for that person (note the similarity with nineteenth-century notions of the multiplicity of causes of infection) since everything was relative (the analytic term is "overdetermined") anyway. Creative writers and the philosophically inclined loved this reasoning, because no matter how bizarre the premise, one could always find some grain of truth somewhere. One can't help but think how fortunate we are that aeronautical engineers, and not artists, design airplanes.

Superior treatment came to be understood as that which the wealthy and the creative community got. Inferior treatment was what those in state hospitals (and places like Washington University) got and was more likely to include something "medical" (e.g., drugs or shock treatment [lobotomies were no longer available in 1966]).

Nonetheless, there were challenges to these notions, and things were beginning to change. As an intern at the Los Angeles County General Hospital in 1965 to 1966, I had the opportunity to learn about research done by a psychiatrist (University of Southern California Medical School was on the campus of Los Angeles County General Hospital) who reported on his research on length of hospital stays (I think his name was Werner

Mendel, but finding USC psychiatry faculty from 1965 proved harder than I'd hoped). He randomly assigned admissions to three different units in the psychiatric division at Los Angeles County General. If admitted (randomly) to unit A, patients stayed for thirty days plus or minus a day or two. If admitted to unit B, patients stayed for sixty days. And in unit C, the stay was around ninety days (Los Angeles County obviously had money in those days). All patients got regular psychotherapy and fairly sophisticated milieu therapy, along with whatever meds the residents/attending felt were necessary. At follow-up, about six to twelve months postdischarge, he reported that there was no way to distinguish those who'd stayed longer from those who had shorter stays. It seemed obvious that factors other than time in hospital treatment played significant roles in outcome, a fact that today we regard as obvious and incontestable.

The community mental health movement of the time also supported the notion that hospitalizations served patients in "crisis" mode but that most other elements of effective therapy could be provided outside of a hospital setting. The purpose of community mental health centers, as originally conceived, was to serve those with major mental illnesses who were returning to the community usually after very long state hospital stays. The new psychotropic drugs made long internments in hospitals unnecessary, but they weren't well as a rule and required ongoing treatment and support.

"Behavior therapy" began to attract attention in the treatment world, developments from academic psychology primarily based on the work of the "behaviorists," like B. F. Skinner, John Watson, and a host of others going back to Pavlov in early-twentieth-century St. Petersburg. Learning to adapt the techniques of Pavlovian and Skinnerian conditioning with animals to human beings was challenging at times, especially when it came to working with adults with "neurotic" problems.

A South African psychiatrist, Joseph Wolpe, attracted the attention of American psychiatrists since he'd reported (through various published reports) apparent good results in working with anxious and depressed adults. Psychiatrist Seymour Halleck reported (in a class at the University of Wisconsin that I attended in 1972) on his experience as a resident at the Menninger Clinic in the late 1950s or early 1960's where Dr. Wolpe had been invited to give a lecture. His theory and techniques were contrary to anything that anyone in the audience had ever heard of or imagined. After Dr. Wolpe had departed the lecture hall, the residents were told to ignore what they'd just heard because the Menninger faculty thought Dr. Wolpe to be a raving psychotic, having made no sense at all (to them).

Another development was the sudden discovery of manic depression after the 1970 introduction of lithium in the United States (again, much earlier in every other modern country) forced a reexamination of a medical model of mental illness. If, in fact, there was something specific about the action of lithium for a particular variety of mental illness, then it became more and more obvious that the brain was indeed relevant in psychiatry, and there was value in knowing what was going on in it. The same process started fifteen years earlier with Thorazine. If antipsychotics were more than just sedatives with a better safety record, then maybe it was time to look at some of our basic assumptions about the causes of mental illness. Maybe the brain was worth studying after all.

Just as the advent of health insurance broadened the base of potential patients treated in the private sector, it also led to concerns about cost, effectiveness, and value for the money. Even in a tax-supported system, like a state university hospital (e.g., University of Illinois, UCLA), questions about value were starting to be asked, and psychoanalytic practices, once thought to be superior, were having trouble justifying their costs.

An example was Madden Mental Health Center in 1972. My contact with Madden came as part of the recruitment of me by Loyola University's medical school to help in developing a child psychiatry training resource. The "geographic full time" contract included being a part-time medical director of Madden's Pavilion 12, a child unit of twenty-four beds for children up to twelve years of age. A parking lot separated Pavilion 12 from the medical school and university hospital.

In the director's office at Madden on day one, the desk was filled with copies of letters to various referral sources regretting the fact that there was no room on the twenty-four-bed child psychiatry unit for the child they wished to refer. The average length of stay on the unit was twenty-two months, which meant that once the unit filled, new admissions had to wait for discharges, which could be many months in the future, as both admissions and discharges became rare. Even after twenty-two months, most of these children continued to require some form of residential care.

At the time, the Orthogenic School at the University of Chicago was seen by some as a model of what the "best" in psychiatric treatment for children should look like. Its famous director, Dr. Bruno Bettelheim, had written a number of books for popular consumption (not peer reviewed), which presumed to explain the causes of child psychiatric disturbances, like autism, and their treatment. It was never quite clear where Dr. Bettelheim was trained and what his qualifications really were, but there was little doubt that he knew a great deal about children and psychoanalytic jargon. He was apparently not a believer in disciplined research or a medical model of illness.

It was unclear whether or not the previous director of Pavilion 12 was a disciple of Dr. Bettelheim, but he was described as dedicated and ethical and had obviously designed a program of treatment that he believed to be of high quality. While they didn't treat many patients per year, it was clear that he believed that those who were treated got the best that taxpayer monies could buy (since this was a state-supported hospital, health insurance was never an issue). Drawing distinctions between active treatment of disorders to effect specific changes within a certain timetable and the treatment of very chronic conditions was not of value here.

In attempting to make these distinctions with differing treatment goals for different patients (now referred to as individualized treatment), the average length of stay dropped from twenty-two months to four months (incredibly long by today's standards, but considered very short-term then). The result was that we were able to treat about six times as many, going from about twelve admits per year to around seventy-two. Was what we did good treatment? There simply were no studies comparing one therapeutic approach to another in this population, so one can never say for sure. Feedback came largely from referral sources whose opinions were that we were at least as effective as in previous years and probably more so, but at one-sixth the cost. We did a follow-up study, which showed that about two-thirds of children were living at home twelve months postdischarge, with about one-third still in some form of residential care (Shearer 1976)

Also during my five years at Madden, another experience brought home the questionable relationship between cost and quality. This one had to do with the treatment of autism at a publicly funded community program. For whatever reason, I was asked to do a report on an autism treatment program on Chicago's southeast side not far from the University of Chicago's Orthogenic School. While not directly affiliated, there was obviously considerable influence in that the treatment approach was very much like that advocated in Dr. Bettelheim's book, The Empty Fortress (1956). Many of the younger staff were students at the University of Chicago and elsewhere, and the more senior staff were or had been in psychoanalysis, which was common at the time. This was 1976, and the children labeled "autistic" were very much autistic since the incidence of autism at that time was estimated to be between one in 2,500 and perhaps at the most one in 1,000. These were very severe cases.

The "Bettelheim approach," based presumably on psychoanalytic theory (meaning that brain function and genetics had nothing at all to do with anything), presumed that autism was a disorder of very traumatic early experience, what he called the "extreme situation." By drifting from a medical/scientific approach, psychoanalysis allowed someone trained in the arts (Bettelheim) to confidently make statements of significant scientific import sans the bother of a scientific education. Bettelheim had spent a few months in a concentration camp prior to immigrating to the United States and felt he'd become an expert on human reactions in extreme situations (Pollak 1997). From there it was a short leap to deciding, and writing papers and books about, the "causes" of autism and schizophrenia (Bettelheim). This is clearly creative speculative science without the bother or the rigor of science.

The program being inspected was based on the Bettelheim "extreme situation" hypothesis. This involved lots of kind and gentle acceptance of whatever behavior the child displayed, and some of these children could be aggressive or were not yet toilet trained. This made for some challenging moments since redirecting a behavior was sometimes seen as rejection of the child, which was the presumed method of autism causation in the first place. Since these children were very autistic and could be identified rather early in life, it meant that they came at a young age and stayed a very long time. The staff were extremely committed and gave a great deal of themselves. The problem with an "extreme situation" hypothesis is that one has to account for and identify an extreme situation. In the absence of Nazis, sadistic SS guards, and concentration camps, one had to conclude that the nice-appearing parents were the creators of the extreme situations that these children had to have experienced. If a parent could cause this much disturbance so early in life, it must have been really bad.

However, the task here was to evaluate effectiveness. Reports by the staff suggested significant progress, and there no doubt was some. If one starts in a program at age three or four and is now age nine or ten, the challenge was to look at how much progress could be attributed to the program and how much to being six years older. The published literature of the time included Leo Kanner's original paper in 1943, from which the term "autistic" was coined (Shearer 1976). These were eleven patients who received no specific-to-autism treatment to speak of but were followed up years later by Leon Eisenberg (Kanner 1943). There was also Michael Rutter's group in England, a group at Indiana University, as well as the series I was personally familiar with at UCLA as a child psychiatry resident at that institution (Eisenberg 1956). That progress was both occurring and in some way related to the treatment program was basically an act of faith with little else to support it.

The UCLA group of autistic children was treated using a behaviorist methodology developed by Dr. Ivar Lovaas. Despite reporting on remarkable language acquisition seen in the films produced at the time about these children, it seemed clear when I saw these children themselves that they were still very autistic, many still barely verbal despite advancing age, and extremely impaired. These were children with something very wrong with their cerebral wiring, and empathy was clearly not going to be the answer, although lack of empathy could clearly make things worse. In the case of autism, psychoanalytic thinking seemed to offer little insight and no hope of viable treatment, Dr. Bettelheim notwithstanding. Dr. Lovaas gave us a model for some kind of educational intervention at least but little help in understanding just what this was.

Once again the relationship between cost and quality was beginning to look very unclear, and the usefulness of analytic theory in designing treatment, at least at the institutional level, was becoming more and more suspect.

The legacy of psychoanalytic ascendancy in psychiatry was in the final analysis (no pun intended) a disunited profession that found it difficult to explain to the public at large, businesses, insurance companies, and government just what it did believe was going on in the human mind generally and in mental illness specifically. It created the belief by some that every aspect of human functioning, from mental illness to the political behavior of nations, could be understood through the analytic process (there could be Freudian interpretations of society alongside Marxist or even Maoist interpretations). It stimulated the development, investigation, and legitimization of various forms of psychotherapy, many of which are used effectively on a daily basis today. The disunity was irremediable, however, and, since nature abhors a vacuum, the "market" took over.

Oddly enough, as he was writing his landmark The Interpretation of Dreams (1900), Freud was also working on another book, which no one (i.e., the general public) knew about until it was finally published in 1953. It was called Project for a Scientific Psychology. In it he attempted to see psychiatry develop in a truly scientific direction, but he clearly saw that the basic science and technology of the time were inadequate to the task. Psychoanalysis is still spoken of in a spirit of profound reverence by many in and out of psychiatry, and its absence in much of today's psychiatry is seen as the cause of the profession's (and society's) troubles. In that vein it continues to bear a canny resemblance to revealed religion.

CHAPTER 11

PSYCHIATRY, HEALTH INSURANCE, AND THE CONCEPT OF MORAL HAZARD

The widespread adoption of health insurance for psychiatric conditions in the mid-1960s and later had a number of interesting consequences. In the five hundred or so years before health insurance, there were private institutions run by the Alexian Brothers and others, and long stays were commonplace since treatment options were limited. The asylum model was in ascendancy since there was basically no alternative to simply taking as much time as necessary for recovery, if indeed recovery was to occur at all. Before psychoanalysis, treatment took many years, but recovery did occur in some patients. With psychoanalysis, recovery still took many years, but there was a belief that now patients had a better understanding of the causes and at least precipitants of their disturbances ("illness" was still an uncomfortable word in these times) and that somehow this knowledge would fortify them against relapse in the future.

In 1946, the film The Snake Pit tried to project an optimistic outlook for the treatment of hospitalized mentally ill patients treated by the new psychoanalytic method, contrasting it with the hopelessness of the psychiatric treatment of the day. It helped popularize the notion that there was a more specific underlying "cause," which the analyst would uncover and, like the surgeon, free the patient of its toxic influence.

The medical model of illness has always focused on outcomes (even if causes remain unknown, which is a problem for most diseases). As reported in chapter 4, Joseph Lister published his results, which documented the dramatic decline in mortality related to his use of sterile technique. In the world of public health, Cuban Dr. Carlos Finlay, in the 1880s, not only identified that yellow fever was transmitted by mosquitoes but actually identified which mosquito, among the many species, was at fault. Proof of Finlay's hypothesis came from the work of Walter Reed and William Gorgas, who eliminated yellow fever from Havana. Gorgas did nothing less than demonstrate the dramatic decline in the incidence of yellow fever and malaria in the Canal Zone between 1905 and 1914. The Mayo brothers published morbidity and mortality rates for a host of different surgical procedures, which were so remarkable that surgeons from all over the world traveled to Rochester, Minnesota, to verify and report on what initially were thought of as possibly faked reports.

In psychiatry, results were not dramatic, but following medical tradition, Emil Kraepelin published on recovery rates and long-term follow-up of hospitalized patients and described the bipolar nature of manic-depressive illness (Kraepelin 1913). With the introduction of electroconvulsive therapy (ECT) in 1938 and the introduction of Thorazine and antidepressants in the 1950s, controlled trials became possible.

It was also at this time in history that some began to question the implicit acceptance of analytic principles in psychiatry. The research of Rosenthal (1971), Kety (1971), and Wender (1974) strengthened the evidence for genetic factors in major mental illness and in alcoholism, and the methodical studies of UCLA professor Philip May at Camarillo State Hospital in California left little doubt regarding the effectiveness of antipsychotic medication in the treatment of schizophrenia (May 1968).

As related in chapter 10, Freud felt analysis had little to offer the mentally ill housed in asylums, and those in analytic training were spending very little time treating hospitalized psychiatric patients. But while the science may have been suspect, the practitioners of psychoanalysis and psychoanalytic therapies were, by and large, ethical.

However, the adoption of psychoanalytic methods in the treatment of large numbers of now-insured patients from middle America quickly resulted in a dramatic expansion of psychiatric bed capacity in the form of venture capital–financed psychiatric hospital companies springing from nowhere to national prominence almost overnight. While the large state institutions were (as of the late 1950s still accounting for 50 percent of all occupied hospital beds in the country) beginning to downsize and achieving shorter lengths of stay, long stays in these new private hospitals, using a long-term treatment model, became a source of significant profit for publicly (and privately) held companies.

By 1975, companies like Psychiatric Institutes of America (PIA), Charter, Community Psychiatric Centers (CPC), and others were building hospitals on seemingly every main street in every town in America. Psychiatry had truly become local, and the "best" treatment somebody else's money could buy became available everywhere. Since the state hospitals were still in existence, uninsured patients could be steered to state-supported facilities, charity care unnecessary. It was win-win for everyone … for a time. Profits were rumored to be at times about 40 percent of gross revenue, which made investing in psychiatric hospitals extremely attractive.

The free market is a wonderful thing, and, in my opinion, it is the basis of most of the wealth on the planet. In general, competition in business results in better quality at the lowest possible prices, encourages innovation, and facilitates the highest standards of living for workers and consumers where productivity is high. As an investor of retirement funds, I expect maximum return on investment since, apart from Social Security, no government agency guarantees my retirement security. The free market even has a place in health care, and innovations that save lives and decrease costs certainly have a place.

However, the free market in health care may be both inappropriate and unnecessarily expensive. In health care there is something called "mission," and it is to look after the health needs of the population of patients (and potential patients) first and foremost. Sometimes conflicts of interest between the needs of the sick and the needs of a health care organization arise. Unfortunately, there exists the risk of creating enterprises specifically designed to extract money from insurance trusts set up with the best intent of helping bring the best care to the employees of industrial organizations or recipients of government sponsored programs. The United States spends more per capita on health care than any other country in the world, and there still are millions with no coverage at all. In selling stock to potential stockholders, the emphasis is on the profit potential and expected "performance" of the company. As an investor, one is not interested in investing (an oxymoron) in charity. One gives to charitable enterprises but does not invest in them in the hope of major return on investment.

Moreover, with broader insurance coverage, health care organizations needed to be motivated by a sense of "ethical stewardship" in order to use the resources of an insurance trust in ways likely to do the best for the greatest number. This concept at times comes into conflict with the performance requirements of a given stock. Between 1966 and 1989 (give or take), there was money to be made in hospital psychiatry, as well as in for-profit medical/surgical hospital ventures. Excesses developed rapidly, and the potential for profit became turbocharged. With dramatic increases in bed capacity, there resulted an increasing need to fill those beds by whatever means modern sales and marketing strategies could devise. Unfortunately, ethical stewardship was not a course doctors took as part of their residency training, and nor did hospital administrators in business schools at that time in history (though now they do).

The difference between a long-term health care ministry and a modern business model is considerable. In the days before health insurance, most, if not all, hospitals charged according to ability to pay. The wealthy paid a lot, and the poor paid nothing, and those in between paid somewhere in between. Since state hospitals were still with us, the plethora of new psychiatric hospitals building nationwide felt they could concentrate on those with health insurance and exclude everyone else. Profits were attractive enough to interest investment bankers who, as part of a business model, are generally not into charity work.

The business model for these new for-profit hospital empires, and the doctors who supported them, was to generate as much revenue as possible in as short a time as possible, and if and when that dried up, go onto something else. Psychiatry today, perhaps dog biscuits tomorrow. Smart investors go where the money is. Even in the for-profit general medical business, there are services that pay well and services that don't. The strategy is to invest heavily in those that pay well and leave the poorly paying to hospitals with "missions" or someone else (government?) to take up the slack.

In the 1970s and later was the rapid development of special education mandates that required schools to develop programs for problematic students who had problems coping with general education and regular classes. The Education for All Handicapped Children Act or Public Law (PL) 94-142 was passed in 1975. It contained a provision requiring disabled students to be placed in a least restrictive environment, allowing maximal exposure to nonimpaired students.

It seemed fortuitous indeed when schools discovered that a psychiatric hospital could keep a problematic student hospitalized for months, relieving the school of an onerous and costly responsibility while giving investors a great return on investment. As a psychiatrist with special training in child/adolescent psychiatry, I, in the 1970s and early 1980s, was often called upon to engage in behavior that the insurers referred to as "morally hazardous" and challenged the principle of "ethical stewardship." Since the dominant model at that time was a long-term one, the unethical nature of keeping patients in the hospital longer than necessary was not always readily apparent. To those actively engaged in hospital work, the charade was obvious. There was simply no one but the attending physician who could make that decision.

For example, the patient was thirteen years old and hospitalized by me sometime in the mid-1970s. Although hospital stays were longer in the 1970s for most of us, there were limits to necessity. The patient was in the hospital for probably about four or five weeks but by the end of March was, in the opinion of our staff, ready to return to school. When the school was contacted to set up a discharge staffing, the school psychologist called back to ask if we would consider keeping the patient until school got out in June. The patient was in eighth grade, and he'd be going to a different school next academic year, so why not? There were only ten more weeks until graduation. The fact that the school psychologist felt comfortable making such a request suggested that this was common practice at many hospitals that the school regularly referred to, and the unspoken message was clearly that if our hospital wished to be considered for referrals, we might wish to reconsider our plans.

Another example comes from my experience serving on the ethics committee of the Illinois Psychiatric Society in the late 1970s or early 1980s. This committee reviewed ethics complaints leveled against psychiatrist members, mostly from patients, or parents of patients, or sometimes spouses or other relatives of patients. One mother filed a complaint against a psychiatrist for not keeping her teenage child in the hospital long enough.

Her son had a very serious psychotic illness but did well with treatment and was discharged after about six or eight weeks in the hospital. The woman argued that other patients in her son's unit seemed much less ill yet were staying three or four months longer on average. She got her information by speaking with the parents of the other teenage patients in her son's unit and felt her son was somehow being shortchanged.

In this case, the ethics committee sided with the doctor. He argued that he was acting ethically by not keeping him in the hospital longer than necessary and questioned the ethics of the hospital and some of his peers who encouraged what he regarded as waste. This was an unusual doctor at this hospital at this time in history and supports the old adage that a good deed seldom goes unpunished.

Since there was no managed care in the 1960s, 1970s, and early 1980s, what treatment a patient got was dictated by whatever the "market" could bear. Surgery by its nature had very specific goals and targets, and pathological examination could, after the fact, verify the "medical necessity" of a procedure. As we discussed in chapter 9, some procedures were questionable and perhaps overused, but the surgeon was paid by the procedure, so there was never any incentive for a surgeon to keep a patient in the hospital longer than absolutely necessary. The incentive was in doing more procedures. In those times, however, patients stayed longer after relatively routine procedures like childbirth and various surgeries. When these were shown to be unnecessary over time, they were quickly abandoned with relatively few complaints by surgeons, although hospitals and sometimes patients were chagrined.

Medical admissions for diagnoses like pneumonia, or cardiac conditions like congestive heart failure, or other infectious processes, usually responded relatively quickly to antibiotics or whatever else was in vogue at the time and insurances could expect admissions to be within a certain range in terms of days in hospital. Many patients thought ill enough to admit in the 1970s for "tests" and to explore obscure and vague symptoms could never be admitted today. Tests are still done, but today more would be done on an outpatient basis. Insurance personnel seemed to understand and accept the necessity of these admissions for the most part. Yes, there were outliers (patients who stayed longer than projected), but they tended to be a predictable percentage of total admissions and didn't vary much from place to place.

In psychiatry it was a different matter altogether. Hospital stays might be incredibly long—perhaps years—and vary greatly depending on location of the hospital. Most insurance reviews, when they occurred, were after the fact. Reading the reasons for remaining in the hospital, reviewers found the explanations baffling; patients were "reliving early trauma" or "working through" issues of abandonment or sibling rivalry or "inferiority complexes" or "low self-esteem." How these issues translated into the need for another year in the hospital was baffling and seemingly incomprehensible to a nonpsychiatrist. More than a few psychiatrists were baffled, as well.

However, Wall Street had discovered that considerable profit rewarded those who wedded themselves to a long-term psychotherapy model of inpatient treatment and catered to the special education needs of friendly school districts. Although insurance in psychiatry (and in health care generally) had not been available for very long, employer-sponsored insurance suddenly began to seem like a God-given right and began to take on a moral dimension. The healing professions had decided that the function of insurance was to pay for whatever (presumably necessary) services we ordered, and it was not the business of insurance to evaluate effectiveness or judge necessity, and that was that. The moral dimension came with the understanding that doctors and hospitals were essentially doing God's work, and any attempt to limit or control costs in any way was regarded as not just unfair but immoral, as well.

By the close of the 1970s, the handwriting was on the wall, but the currently profitable strategy was to ignore handwriting on walls. While there were notable variations in surgery early on (e.g., hysterectomies and tonsillectomies), insurers found it easier to control these practices by consensus and follow-up research. In psychiatry the variability in practice was much broader than in other branches of medicine. Follow-up studies on effectiveness (like Dr. Mendel at USC) were either ignored or explained in incomprehensible language and varied dramatically by location. Alex Spadoni, mentioned in chapter 1, has surveyed hospitals in Illinois for years. He reported thirty years ago that lengths of stay in hospitals north of Interstate 80 (Chicago and suburbs) were consistently much longer than those south of that highway. Maybe there was more serious mental illness north of Interstate 80, or more investor-owned hospitals. There would be more.

As costs mounted and insurers began to push back, it became apparent that the systems we'd come to know and love were unsustainable. The only question was what changes were coming, and how quickly would they come? In the 1970s and early 1980s, Blue Cross of Illinois (and others) began challenging these very long stays by threatening nonpayment in some cases. Hospitals countered by threatening lawsuits, arguing breach of contract since the business of insurance was (in theory) to insure and pay for, but not dictate, treatment. At first, the suing hospitals won some of these cases, which gave some of them a false sense of righteousness and invulnerability that comes with the belief that one is doing God's own work—perhaps a modern version of the ancient Alexians' "imitation of Christ" but with better returns on investment.

It was false and short-lived security. Instead of trying to work with the insurers for the sake of both patients and ourselves to find some reasonable path, doctors and hospitals derided insurers as profit mongers (our motives were pure, theirs weren't), and we basically went to war. Since most private insurance is employer-based, and health insurance was having a major impact on bottom lines, insurers fought back by encouraging employers to cut psychiatric benefits. Additionally, breach-of-contract issues were relatively easily dealt with by simply rewriting contracts. The inevitable groundwork was being laid for what was later to become known as "managed care."

National (American Psychiatric Association) and local (Illinois Psychiatric Society) psychiatric professional organizations were, naturally, very concerned about these changes. However, professional organizations are made up of doctors of various persuasions and outlooks and found it difficult to be flexible since that would mean offending one kind of practitioner or another. The underlying, not always articulated issue during these times was who would control how psychiatric benefits were designed in employee benefit plans.

An analogy might be the National Rifle Association (NRA) but without the legislative clout. The NRA probably has some, possibly many, members who would be willing to compromise on things like the size of magazine clips and the open availability of assault weapons, but there are members who manufacture and sell assault weapons with super-sized magazine clips, so the NRA gives up nothing and apparently has the legislative clout to get away with it.

In psychiatry we weren't so lucky. Our professional organizations could not take positions on issues where it looked like we were giving in regarding limits on inpatient days (assault weapons) or on outpatient visits (magazine clips), so we basically did nothing. As we will see, professional organizations were relatively impotent, and the "market" ultimately did the dictating.

In the 1970s, there was no such thing as "utilization review," now a large department at all hospitals, psychiatric and otherwise. Prior to the coming of managed care, the local medical societies began to feel that they should try to play some role in mediating insurance disputes, which were increasing in frequency and in ill will. Some insurance companies sought out objective advice on how to respond to some of these claims, being puzzled by psychiatric terminology and practice. To its credit, the Illinois Psychiatric Society put together an insurance committee composed of psychiatrists of various persuasions, including three practicing psychoanalysts (the committee had nine members). The committee met monthly and reviewed cases referred by various insurance companies for no charge (incomprehensible by today's standards). This was seen as a kind of community service obligation of a professional society in the interest of developing standards, and educating insurance companies in the interest of patients and ourselves.

These were meant to be as objective as possible, and we did not see ourselves as charged with the task of defending our members against the insurers. The future of the profession seemed more important than the futures of individual members. (There was a lawsuit of hospital against insurance company in one of our cases, so I had the opportunity to testify in one of these early lawsuits on the East Coast.)

We found ourselves agreeing with the insurers much more often than we thought we would. We came to agree that many of the cases we reviewed saw huge expenditures with questionable outcomes based on idiosyncratic thinking and often lacking objective evidence for many of the treatment decisions. What was surprising was that, despite our varying orientations, we were able to agree on the great majority of cases. Perhaps the insurance companies were sending us the most egregious cases, over which we had little disagreement. We were never sure. What we could say for sure was that our work did little to influence psychiatric society issues, and soon afterward organizations came into being that did what we did but for a fee. Cases referred for review, of course, increased dramatically and, ultimately, required full-time professional review organizations.

Outpatient office-based treatment was also an issue. Some patients were in treatment for years, and trying to explain why was often challenging. Psychoanalytic and psychotherapy jargon was difficult for those educated outside of a particular school of analysis or therapy to make sense of. This lent credence to insurer beliefs that psychiatric treatment was unpredictable (actuaries believe in statistical probabilities) and, therefore, uninsurable. Many problems seemed like "problems in living" rather than illness and issues everyone had to deal with. With this view virtually everyone was a potential patient, so some populations turned out to be very high utilizers (e.g., highly skilled workers or professionals at major companies).

While I served on the psychiatric society's ethics committee one year, a married couple came in to complain about a breach of confidentiality by a member psychiatrist. The alleged breach is not germane to this discussion, but the couple had recently moved to Chicago from another city. They had been in therapy, individually and as a couple, for years. Over the years they had lived in several cities and with each move had not only bought a new home but scouted out new therapists. They didn't see therapy as having a beginning or an end but as a perpetual process that they assumed they were entitled to by virtue of having a job with insurance benefits. Diagnosis was usually irrelevant except that insurance wouldn't pay the bills without one. Therapy seemed to have no goal other than to try to find a goal. Woody Allen would have understood perfectly, but insurance companies saw this practice as a "moral hazard" of insurance in mental health.

In Chicago, psychiatric residents interested in psychoanalysis were expected to get bank loans, and a local bank agreed to finance. One year at a national meeting, I met a resident training in Washington, DC, who moonlighted at St. Elizabeths (psychiatric) Hospital, a federal facility. Working a few evening hours a week entitled him to full federal health insurance benefits, which he used to fund his analysis. In Chicago, this was considered a training expense. In DC, it was covered by federal health insurance plans. These are the kinds of outpatient issues that made funding psychiatric treatment suspect in the eyes of insurers.

CHAPTER 12

ALEXIAN BROTHERS MEDICAL CENTER, 1972–1999

My first contact with Alexian Brothers was in 1972 as a corollary of employment at Loyola's medical school and Madden Mental Health Center, although I didn't become a member of the medical staff until 1977. The psychiatry units at Alexian Brothers were clinical teaching sites (as was Madden Mental Health) for the Loyola residents of the time, who included among them Dr. Gregory Teas. The new chair in psychiatry that year at Alexian Brothers was C. Buckland (Cork) Thomas, who had just arrived from the Monroe Clinic in Wisconsin. Dr. Thomas's recruitment was something of a joint venture between Loyola and Alexian Brothers in the way that mine was between Loyola and Madden Mental Health Center. Dr. Thomas did not have an active private practice at Alexian Brothers, but he did have administrative duties as the chair in psychiatry, and he had teaching and supervision responsibilities through Loyola. Dr. Thomas was an unusual chair given the time since all other chairs were actively practicing private physicians and the chairmanship only part-time. Even the medical director of the hospital at the time, Dr. Sheldon Cohen, was part-time.

The hiring of Dr. Thomas may have been symptomatic of the acrimony between administration and medical staff at Alexian Brothers in the years between 1968 (the hospital only opened in 1966) and 1977. This clash ultimately resulted in a variety of Illinois case law decisions involving hospitals and medical staffs and what each could and could not do with one another.

Since I hadn't joined the staff until May 1977, it was difficult to understand all of the issues involved, and I wasn't aware of the conflict until I'd been on staff for some time. I'm told it was a highly contentious environment.

While the department of psychiatry is usually not an area of exceptional conflict and disagreement (in contrast to a department like surgery, given the multiplicity of privileges and more intense competition), the president of the medical staff during several years of this contentious decade was a psychiatrist who was a very strong advocate for the medical staff as a whole.

Without getting into the issue of who was right and who was wrong, the Brothers and the hospital board of directors apparently felt dissatisfied with the quality and practice of at least some of the medical staff, which led them to institute the hired chair model. This represented something of a deviation from what was commonly practiced at community hospitals, which was the election of department chairs by the medical staff sans interference by administration. Today it's not particularly unusual for community hospitals and medical centers to have chairs appointed by a hospital's board of directors after a search committee has done its work by interviewing candidates and making its recommendations to the board. In the 1960s and 1970s, this was less common at the community hospital level but common practice at university hospitals and teaching centers for centuries.

The function of a department chair was to represent the members of the department in question with the position of president of the medical staff representing the entire medical staff to the hospital board. A chair elected exclusively by a vote of the department members implies a physician respected by his or her colleagues with the expectation of representing their interests. When this model works well, communication between physicians and administration flows easily both ways. The interests of patients are often well served since physicians are on the front line and can often see quickly what is and what is not effective for their patients, and needed changes can be quickly implemented. Obvious quality issues that come to the attention of a department chair are addressed appropriately and in a timely manner. Maverick physicians are counseled in a collegial manner and brought into line by the chair or colleagues in the department.

In this most traditional model, the physician is a client or "customer" of the hospital, in that the patients "belong" to the physician who elects to bring the patient to the hospital for its nursing and/or diagnostic services. In a large metropolitan area with many different hospitals, physicians unhappy with the services at one hospital can easily steer his or her patients to some other. This model is potentially ideal, in that it maximizes physician involvement in the hospital.

But it didn't always work. Some physicians (then and now) felt that what's good for the doctor must be, ipso facto, good for the patient, and in the majority of cases that is probably true. But the majority of cases aren't the problem. As with most issues of medical quality, it's the minority of cases that distinguish high- versus low-quality medical care, along with, at times, perverse economic incentives. Moreover, in day-to-day practice, it was very difficult to sanction a colleague if that doctor was a significant source of referrals to the hospital or to one's own practice, depending on specialty.

The hired chair model was meant to continue the traditional duties of a chair to represent his or her department members vis-à-vis administration, but the primary duty, as the board saw it, was to advocate for the patient and the community even if potentially averse to the interests of the department members. In the days before quality oversight committees were in full operation, there was a tendency to notice questionable practices only when something went wrong. Modern concepts of quality control dictate that the hospital and the medical staff intervene before something goes wrong wherever possible. In the current environment, doctors are regaled with discussions about "best practices," through which research and internal departmental review is expected to identify which practices are, in fact, truly best. Like so many things, that is easier said than done. Most doctors see themselves as at least the equal of their peers and don't take criticism or sanction lightly, making the role of chair, especially in the 1970s and 1980s (and today), highly challenging.

Dr. Thomas did not stay as chair very long. The reason may have had something to do with the medical staff's natural suspicion of nonpracticing chairs of departments and possibly saw his appointment as portent of things to come in other departments (i.e., domination in some way by administration or a medical school affiliation). There may have been other more personal reasons on Dr. Thomas's part. Whatever the reason, the next chair beginning in 1974 was like the other hired chairs, part-time. His name was Michael Rogers, MD.

I came to know Dr. Rogers through his participation on the teaching staff in Loyola's psychiatric residency training program, and he eventually prevailed upon me to join the staff at Alexian Brothers Medical Center in 1977. The faculty at Loyola, at least in psychiatry, had a significant influence on practice at Alexian Brothers, even when the teaching affiliation diminished in the mid-2000s. Residents at Loyola in the early 1970s included: Drs. Greg Teas, Charles Hillenbrand, Barry Rabin, Roger Konwal, and Philip Janicak. All but Dr. Janicak practiced at Alexian Brothers in the 1970s and later. Other residents included: Dr. Robert Zadylak, who eventually became chief medical officer at the Illinois Masonic Medical Center in Chicago; Dr. Daniel Anzia, who later replaced Dr. Patrick Staunton upon his retirement as chair in psychiatry at Lutheran General; Dr. Vince Sackett, who became chair at Central DuPage Hospital; Dr. Jack Curns, who became chair at St. Therese Hospital in Waukegan; and Dr. Mark Sinibaldi at Little Company of Mary Hospital in the Palos Hills area of the south suburbs.

Faculty at Loyola included, in addition to Michael Rogers: Dr. Alex Spadoni, who was psychiatry chair at St. Joseph's in Joliet and a member of the state of Illinois's hospital licensing board; and Dr. Patrick Staunton, district director for region 2 (Chicago area) of the Illinois Department of Mental Health and later chair at Lutheran General Hospital in Park Ridge. Dr. Staunton was for many years chair of the ethics committee of the American Psychiatric Association; Dr. Cullen Schwemmer was residency training director who in 1976 became department chair at Good Samaritan Hospital in Downers Grove. Dr. Robert DeVito was superintendent at Madden Mental Health Center and for a time chief of Illinois's Department of Mental Health. Barry Rabin became psychiatry chair at St. Joseph's newly built hospital in Elgin in 1975. Dr. Janicak had a distinguished career as professor of psychiatry at the University of Illinois and published his own textbook of psychopharmacology. Dr. Janicak was one of the original researchers in transcranial magnetic stimulation (rTMS), in collaboration with the psychiatry department at Alexian Brothers in the mid-1990s.

What seemed to differentiate Loyola from the other programs in Chicago at the time was its stronger emphasis on a medical model in psychiatry (which was not seen as an asset among local programs) with the active encouragement of the hospital as a legitimate locus of practice in psychiatry. It was the treatment model adopted by Alexian Brothers, as it was at most of the psychiatric divisions of general hospitals in the Chicago area. There were few, if any, Loyola people involved in any appreciable way with the major for-profit psychiatric hospitals in the 1970s and 1980s. This most likely was not accidental.

It was Alex Spadoni and Patrick Staunton, both active in teaching at Loyola, who were influential in my career by their encouraging of active involvement in the Illinois Psychiatric Society on various committees, as president in 1986, and as a hospital surveyor for the Hospital Licensing Division of the Illinois Department of Public Health in the late 1970s and early 1980s. It was their strong opinion that the lack of what I earlier called "ethical stewardship" by the psychiatric hospital industry would be disastrous for the profession and the patients whom we served. It was their opinion that the Wall Street game plan was to make as much money as possible and then, when no longer profitable, leave (there seemed to be no commitment to either patients or profession). That, oddly enough, is exactly what happened.

As a hospital licensing surveyor, because of my child/adolescent subspecialty, I was assigned to survey the hospitals that had the largest populations of patients under the age of eighteen. These hospitals were usually the very large for-profit institutions. I was surprised to see that hospitals with 150 to over 200 beds had fewer admissions per year than we did at Alexian Brothers, with 55 beds. It seemed clear that as long as insurance companies continued to fund very long hospital stays in psychiatry, they would survive. However, unless these large, mostly for-profit hospitals had some strategic plan they weren't talking about (other than suing insurers) by mid-1980, their demise seemed only a matter of time. Just how much time it would take and whether we could survive in the meantime were issues of great importance to us at Alexian Brothers.

But, as insurance contracts were being rewritten and the concept of concurrent (while in hospital) review continued to gather strength, costs continued to escalate dramatically. As businesses began looking seriously at how to control escalating health care costs, managed care began looking more and more attractive to those who were paying the bills. Managed care was threatening to all doctors at this time, but we in psychiatry felt especially vulnerable because of our feeling that there was, in fact, widespread abuse, and care in psychiatry seemed more "discretionary" to employers who paid for health insurance.

An organization appeared at about this time in history (late 1970s and early 1980s) called the American Association of General Hospital Psychiatrists. This was an organization, one of whose main purposes was to attempt to counter the domination of inpatient psychiatry by the large for-profit hospital companies. The local branch was the Illinois Association of General Hospital Psychiatrists, whose members were those like-minded souls who felt that psychiatry's place was as part of a medical setting in a not-for-profit environment. Dr. Teas and I were active in that organization, as were many of the Loyola faculty and graduates who practiced in the general hospital environment. Our major belief was that long stays in the hospital were no longer supportable on scientific grounds (by the late 1970s) though still practiced widely. Dr. Spadoni's reports for the Illinois Department of Public Health and the Illinois Hospital Association showed the dramatic differences in length of stay depending on whether the Illinois psychiatric hospital was north or south of Interstate 80.

In May 1977, I formally joined the staff at Alexian Brothers as part of a decision to transition into the world of private practice, encouraged strongly by Dr. Rogers. I'd also joined a group headed by Dr. Barry Rabin in Elgin earlier in 1977 but decided to concentrate my activities in the Elk Grove area in 1978 when offered the administrative post of director of the alcohol treatment unit at Alexian Brothers under Michael Rogers. Dr. Rogers had very strong feelings about "ethical stewardship" of health benefits, and that view extended to ethical behavior of physicians in general. This eventually got him into conflict with some members of the staff who preferred a more laissez-faire style of leadership.

Whether it had anything to do with his leadership style or not would be difficult to say, but as a student in Ireland, before immigrating to the United States, his college sport was boxing. He was difficult to intimidate both personally and professionally since he was an avid reader of professional literature and always very current. It was also his opinion that ethical conduct by members of his department was a right all patients were entitled to experience. When, in his opinion, such ethical conduct was found lacking, he felt obligated as department chair to sanction wrongdoers, and he did. In one such case the charges facing one department member were rather serious and had significant career implications for the doctor accused. At Alexian Brothers, the department chairs were not elected by department members (as mentioned earlier), and their principal charge was to protect patients first.

Under the hospital's bylaws (that body of legalisms outlining the rights and obligations of the medical staff, some of which had so recently been decided in court), the accused wrongdoer had the right to have whatever sanction imposed by the department chair reviewed by the medical executive committee. Unfortunately, the committee did not support Dr. Rogers's proposed sanction for what the committee felt was insufficient evidence. Dr. Rogers could produce no witnesses willing to testify to the alleged unethical conduct, and medical staff members, not being employees of the hospital, had rights to due process. Unfortunately, patients will often complain about a physician's behavior, but when the time comes to go public, they refuse to testify, depending on the nature of the complaint. Since there had been more than one complaint about this particular physician, Rogers felt he had no choice but to do the right thing, as he saw it, and took the medical executive committee's decision as a "no confidence" vote on himself (which I do not believe it was). He resigned while then recommending me for his position.

This was January 1979. Managed care did not exist at that time, but the various insurers were beginning to erect barriers to unmanaged care in the form of denials of payment in cases they thought did not meet "medical necessity" guidelines they were attempting to implement.

By 1984, managed care contracting for various medical services was an evolving potential and much talked about but not yet a fact of daily life. Denials in psychiatry had become an issue in some cases, and some hospitals had chosen the lawsuit as a defensive strategy. However, it was anyone's guess what the future held and how it would evolve. The Chicago medical/surgical hospital market was large (more than fifty hospitals), and contracting with large health plans and/or large employers looked like a possibility as a strategy for controlling medical costs generally, not just in psychiatry.

At this point Alexian Brothers entered into a seventeen-hospital consortium spread geographically over the Chicago metropolitan area. It became known as the Health First Network. Some of these hospitals had psychiatric services, and some did not. For insurance carriers and employers alike, psychiatry was something of an enigma, a kind of Pandora's box, out of which actuaries seemed unable to predict utilization to any useful degree, making the risk seem uninsurable. Medical colleagues saw psychiatrists, especially psychoanalytically oriented psychiatrists, as an alien race that spoke a strange and unintelligible language completely without utilization parameters—unlike surgeons, for example.

Therefore, it seemed that if psychiatry at Alexian Brothers and other hospitals in the network were going to play any role at all in the contracting process, we were going to have to make ourselves credible and develop a degree of predictability, or be bypassed as impractical. Alexian Brothers had a number of psychiatrists interested in finding a way to make psychiatric benefits insurable since by now managed care was looming large as a force to be reckoned with. Unless one had been living under a rock for the previous ten years, it was our opinion that we needed to be proactive in developing a managed care strategy.

We decided to develop a network within a network with credible standards of utilization review. This meant minimizing risk for the consortium as a whole and would involve going "at risk" ourselves. Of the seventeen hospitals in the Health First Network, perhaps eight or nine had psychiatric services. Since these were all general hospitals often led by a number of Loyola faculty and trainees, the operating philosophies were more alike than different, even in facilities without Loyola-trained personnel. In 1985, this psychiatry-only network was incorporated and was in place to compete for contracts associated with the Health First organization. As it turned out, the very first managed care contracts inked by the Alexian Brothers Medical Center were in psychiatry, a move some compared to making a compact with the devil. We opined that we would have to deal with managed care (the devil) or ultimately go out of business. Those early contracts served as models for later managed care contracting for the hospital as a whole, according to Mark Frey, the current president of the Alexian Health System, about whom more will be said later in this chapter.

Obviously not everyone in 1985 agreed with the Alexian vision of the brave new world to come. In fact, psychiatric hospital construction moved forward with undiminished vigor. In 1988, a new 95-bed hospital was built in Hoffman Estates. It was built by a group of investors, some of whom were psychiatrists. It was called Woodland Hospital and was soon acquired by a large for-profit hospital chain known as Hospital Corporation of America (HCA), which had earlier acquired the general hospital a few hundred yards to the west. About six miles down Barrington Road, in

Streamwood, another hospital was under construction. A for-profit chain called Community Psychiatric Centers (CPC) was building the 100-bed facility. Directly across the street from the HCA/Woodland Hospital, a certificate of need (CON) was approved for yet another hospital, this time by the large Charter Hospital Corporation, at 80 beds. The field was getting very crowded indeed, although the Charter facility was never built since things were changing rapidly. And if the field wasn't getting crowded enough, a 100-bed addiction treatment hospital had been built during the late 1980s less than one hundred yards from Woodland Hospital. It was the creation of investor-owned Addiction Recovery Centers of America (ARC). Suddenly there were 375 new beds in the neighborhood, including the 80 beds from Charter not yet started.

As proof of the adage that anything is possible in Illinois if there's enough money behind it, yet another 140-bed hospital was approved through the legislative process in Springfield. Apparently the investors who owned a hospital outside New York, called Four Winds, felt Chicago was ripe for what they referred to as a "high end" facility, which would specialize in the long-term treatment of the "seriously mentally ill." In order to get a CON, testimony had to be brought to bear to show that yet another facility was needed in the Chicago area.

Imagine our surprise at how much political support came from every corner and crevice of Illinois. Even though this was to be a high-end facility like the one ostensibly serving the New York City area, support came from a variety of local mental health centers designed to serve the uninsured. They seemed to be strange bedfellows but testified that Illinois needed to have such a hospital to serve "the unmet needs of the chronically mentally ill," presumably with longer-term, "restorative" therapy (which was not further defined but, we thought, one of those things that we'd presumably recognize when we saw it). It billed itself as somehow different, but to most of us it was yet another large, for-profit psychiatric hospital.

The project went through, of course, to the chagrin of those who didn't understand the nature of politics in Illinois. There must have been the expectation of considerable return on investment considering the impressive support this new hospital had orchestrated. The hospital officially opened in 1990. It was called Four Winds, Chicago.

At first, all went as planned. In addition to all these new beds, there were still 180 beds at Forest Hospital, 99 at Lutheran General, and 36 each at Northwest Community and St. Joseph's in Elgin, with Elmhurst, Glendale Heights, and Central DuPage adding at least another 150. One had to suppose that everyone thought they would be the likely survivors. Obviously we all could not be.

Four Winds Hospital, at least relative to Alexian Brothers, was not local. It was in the suburb of Lemont, which is about forty miles south of where we are, although supported politically by a local community mental health center in Arlington Heights. Within days of its opening, as I remembered it, an item appeared in a local newspaper about a securities and exchange issue related to the parent company of this new hospital. I was unable to find the newspaper article while doing research for this publication but was able to find the text of the lawsuit filed in the US District Court in Colorado on August 24, 1992. It cited American Health Properties (AHP) and its officers. AHP at that time owned or operated ten acute care hospitals, five psychiatric hospitals, and six rehabilitation hospitals.

By 1991, managed care was beginning to have some impact on hospital utilization. The suit against AHP by some of its stockholders alleged that by March 1992, the stock price was being artificially inflated by deliberately concealing from investors the abysmal performance of three of the psychiatric hospitals. Reports filed by AHP with the Securities and Exchange Commission were allegedly falsified, giving investors the impression they could expect a dividend of about $2.65 per share and had from 1988 to 1991 experienced a compound annual growth rate of 8 percent. Earnings for the second quarter of 1992 were reported on July 16 to be at 54 cents per share, but on August 17, it was announced that the 54 cents rate had to be "restated," and there was, in fact, a loss of $2.07 per share due to the write-down of the value of the psychiatric hospitals, which came to a tidy $45 million. The suit alleged that the CEO, CFO, and chairman of the board were "insiders" who concealed these facts until they could dispose of their own stock at the inflated prices, which had been based on falsified earnings reports.

Four Winds later changed the name of the hospital to Rock Creek but was never able to ethically find enough patients to make it a profitable undertaking. Instead, hospital administrators apparently concocted elaborate schemes with willing local doctors to admit to the hospital disabled residents from local nursing homes covered by Medicare and Medicaid with flimsy justification. One doctor accepted, according to the *Chicago Tribune's* April 18, 2010, article, "more than $500,000 in kickbacks to steer vulnerable patients. Prosecutors described the scope of the bribes as 'extraordinary.'" Of course, US taxpayers ended up paying the bills. When Rock Creek eventually closed in 2002, the hospital owed Medicare somewhere between $5 million and $17 million, according to a Chicago Tribune article of July 19, 2010.

At Alexian Brothers in 1988, our own survival was certainly not guaranteed by any means. With all the sophisticated local competition from national companies, the issue of continuing or leaving the psychiatric market at least merited some discussion since survival, at least at that time, seemed problematic. We know that at least Charter had made some kind of offer for the Alexian psychiatric assets, and administration was giving it consideration (Charter had won a CON for a new hospital in Hoffman Estates at the time, but CPC and what became Columbia/HCA were already under construction. Given the competition, it made sense for Charter to try to buy into an existing operation).

It was at that time that Dr. Greg Teas and I met with the health system's corporate leadership, who were Dean Grant, James Sances, and Bruce Fisher, to make our case for survival and gave our opinion that neither Charter nor any of the other major for-profit companies were going to survive the managed care onslaught that we saw as inevitable. Our problem was that we couldn't say how quickly the inevitable was going to arrive or how successfully the for-profits could or would want to compete for relatively lower-paying managed care business. Our belief was that the profit requirements (and length-of-stay requirements) of those organizations would make them uncompetitive, and we had just inked our first managed care contract (with Cigna), which seemed to be going well. Their response was that they hoped we knew what we were talking about, but then Alexian Brothers retained control of its psychiatric assets, and Charter, by the way, went out of business about nine years later.

Since it looked like we were going to stay in business, it was time to become a bit more sophisticated in our operations. We felt we needed a more competitive edge. Our psychiatric division (at the Niehoff Pavilion) was housed in a cheaply built facility. The Four Seasons nursing home had sustained several very heavy snowfalls in the winter of 1979 and had not only damaged the roof but also, because of massive heavy snow that stayed frozen for several months, compromised the entire structure. The Illinois Department of Public Health inspections suggested that it would not continue to meet code for patient habitation much longer. However, this did not seem to be an opportune time to ask the Brothers to build a new building.

Our chief operating officer (COO) in 1988 and 1990 was Lee Domanico, who agreed with the psychiatrists, like myself and Dr. Teas, that we at Alexian Brothers were not well positioned to compete with the plethora of new psychiatric hospitals opening in the area. Lee decided to take a look at how our competition operated by visiting a Charter hospital operated by a friend of his in Las Vegas. He came back with a plan to shore up our weaknesses and began by looking at the intake process.

The question to be answered here was how does a patient get into our hospital? The answer was not very easily. We had no dedicated intake personnel. We were a general hospital, and all patients admitted here came either by the request of a physician, in our case a psychiatrist calling admissions and ordering a bed, or through the emergency department, commonly referred to as the ER. Depending on how busy the ER doctors were at the moment a potential patient arrived, our patients could be viewed as, at best, merely annoying or, at worst, unworthy of the space and time they took up while the doctor dealt with the other more "deserving" patients. Alcoholics or drug addicts in withdrawal, or severely intoxicated, were especially unwelcome by virtue of a certain moral taint associated with these behaviors, although they could be highly compromised medically. In fairness to several of the ER doctors, many patients were indeed well treated, but it was hit or miss. If, like many acutely ill psychiatric patients, they were not always well behaved, there could be some tense moments, to say the least.

Mr. Domanico instituted changes that made coming to the ER less onerous for both hospital staff and patients. Mental health professionals became part of the ER staff and relieved the doctors of some of the time-consuming history taking and helped with interviewing relatives or police if they were involved. It became, for the most part, a kinder, gentler experience for patients.

Lee also agreed that, at 55 beds, we were large enough to be considered worthy of more administrative time than the director of nursing (DON) for the hospital could give us since she was generally taken up with medical/surgical issues in this 400-bed community hospital. We had a competent head nurse in psychiatry, but she focused on internal day-to-day operations and still had to run all the important decisions through the DON. This turned out to be very inefficient and tended to delay implementation of new ideas or programs.

While the psychiatrists at Alexian Brothers were firm believers that psychiatry belonged in a medical environment, we also understood that, as just one of many divisions in the hospital, the DON was not going to be able to provide the administrative leadership we needed to compete, and the doctors, including myself, had neither the time nor the business expertise to manage what was a rather large, competitive business operation. A decision was made to look for (most likely) a nonnurse administrator for our division who would still report to the director of nursing but had much more administrative flexibility in decision-making and in dealing with competitive business issues.

A search firm was hired and a national search for an administrative chief of psychiatry undertaken. Of the candidates sent to us, all had been in some administrative position more or less similar to the position being offered. These were seemingly competent candidates with credible management experience in a hospital or mental health center setting. Most were psychologists or psychiatric social workers. Those coming from a mental health center background had little experience in a hospital environment and, if hired, would require some time to learn to function in a medical environment. It is a very different world. Those who had experience working in a hospital environment would have a shorter learning curve.

However, we were hoping to find someone who understood that we were about to embark on a mission for our very survival in the face of what looked like formidable competition from two recently opened psychiatric hospitals, a third waiting to break ground not very far from us, and a recently opened 100-bed addictions hospital, all within nine miles (very close by outer suburban standards) of our front door. Possibly because we were small and relatively unknown, the candidates were disappointing and didn't seem to have any kind of strategy or vision for dealing with the

Anthony M D'Agostino, MD

brave new world we were anticipating in mental health care (and medicine generally). They seemed to understand internal operations well, but we were hoping for something resembling a strategic vision given the challenges.

The search firm got no fees this time around since all candidates seemed unsuitable, and waiting for more of the same seemed a waste of everyone's time. The exercise was useful, however, in that it stimulated us to focus our thinking about what we were looking for in a person in this position and helped us realize that we, in fact, had who we were looking for already employed at the hospital. His name was Mark Frey. Up to that point, administration had not seriously considered him as a candidate.

The reason was probably that, apart from the DON for the hospital and the chief nurse for psychiatry, no one else in administration knew much about him. It was, after all, a 400-bed hospital with over 2,400 employees with psychiatry housed in a separate building across a busy road from the main hospital, with little, if any, staff overlap.

Mark ran the adolescent program, which was quietly successful and very tightly run. Doctors who admitted adolescents knew him well and had great respect for his administrative abilities, but not all doctors worked with adolescents. He was demanding of his staff and occasionally abrasive, but they all seemed to respect him. He was, for the most part, approachable. He wasn't afraid to take on the DON or the doctors when he felt they were wrong or not doing their jobs as well as they should, which created the impression of a strong leader. He took seriously every assignment given him. Those who worked under him would later remember him as the one who was vocal in his complaints about those who managed the hospital as a whole and implied he could do it better. The difference between Mark Frey and the millions of middle managers who daily say the same thing, as time would later demonstrate, is he actually could.

When he was hired in 1977, he had a degree in philosophy, which somehow didn't fit him since he came across as organized and practical and didn't seem to fit the philosophy-major stereotype. Between 1977 and 1990, he worked full-time but continued his education by first getting a master's degree in psychiatric social work since more clinical education seemed appropriate. He then went on to law school. It was unclear if he ever seriously thought about practicing law, but he always felt there were too many things he didn't know enough about, and he'd explain his law school investment as a kind of exercise in the development of, in his words, "disciplined thinking."

It also occurred to him that in the hierarchical world of the medical/ hospital environment, advanced degrees and "disciplined thinking" were important for serious advancement. He worked harder than most everyone else yet made time for schooling and family, having had his three children born in these years. If he had a failing, it was a certain inability to understand why everyone he worked with didn't work as hard as he did. The result, however, was raised expectations and better performance overall.

We were hoping for someone with both competitive instincts and business smarts, and with a little practice, he managed both. He was born with competitive instincts. He acquired business smarts, but he was a fast learner. As adolescent program chief, he knew what was going on not only inside our building but outside in the community, as well. He had an appreciation for issues related to schools and parents and everything else that went on in the outside world that affected us in the hospital. He was in touch with the realities of the changing business environment as it affected his program. He was insightful enough to know what he didn't know and blessed with an aptitude for quick recognition of the relevant issues in problems or situations demanding resolution. He was tactful in situations requiring tact and could be tough in situations demanding toughness. He got things done, no excuses.

Lee Domanico hired Mr. Frey into this newly created position in 1990. It turned out to be perhaps the most important decision affecting the future of psychiatry at Alexian Brothers apart from the Alexian Brothers' decision to purchase the HCA psychiatric hospital building in 1999.

Despite all the hospitals opening around us, we managed to hold our own, though the other hospitals did well also, at least at first. Shortly after hiring Mr. Frey, Lee Domanico left Alexian Brothers for a CEO position at Mercy Hospital in Chicago (the oldest continuously operating hospital in Chicago dating to 1850, mentioned in chapter 3). In his place came Pat Paulson in the COO position (not to be confused with Pat Paulsen, a deadpan comedian who appeared on the Smothers Brothers TV show in the late 1960s and did political satire).

Mark made several initiatives right away. Having worked at the hospital for the past thirteen years in a mostly administrative position, he didn't need much time to familiarize himself with our position in the psychiatric community and could start right in with ideas he felt needed to be implemented. In 1995, the private practice developed by Dr. Teas and me, Behavioral Medicine Associates, merged with the hospital. Greg remained as medical director of the practice and I medical director (or chair) of the psychiatry department. That worked out well enough to continue today as the Alexian Brothers Outpatient Group Practice, now with about eighteen psychiatrists.

Some initiatives didn't work as well. In the 1990s, the medical/psychiatric world was changing quickly, but it wasn't always easy to see what was coming around the next corner. "Carve outs" were the talk of the times, and concerns about being able to compete for and manage capitation contracts "carved out" of a general medical/surgical health plan were part of everyday conversation. Trying to anticipate the future, we made an attempt to partner with a large local outpatient practice with multiple locations. That ultimately didn't work for two reasons: large insurers proved unwilling to turn over very much of that business to local groups, choosing instead to develop their own internal capacities to manage psychiatric care, and there were too many "equal" partners. Inherent differences in corporate cultures made it difficult to achieve consensus on what to do, when to do it, and for what reasons. We lacked what the military would refer to as "unity of command." Some ventures are best accomplished with a single vision rather than multiple competing visions. Partnership, normally an Alexian corporate value, didn't work in this particular situation.

While we had our status as a separate division within the hospital, we were still under the administrative oversight of the director of nursing. Again there were similarities and differences in how we operated versus the rest of the hospital, which, in Mr. Frey's view, limited his ability to act quickly and innovate. Pat Paulson proved to be an important mentor for Mr. Frey by encouraging him to learn how the hospital as a whole operated. Mr. Frey has always spoken appreciatively of that opportunity. Mr. Paulson appreciated Mr. Frey's extraordinary talents and eventually supported his bid for greater autonomy, and psychiatry soon became a separate division reporting directly to the CEO.

Between when he was hired in 1990 and when he left in 1997, despite the depredations of managed care in psychiatry, we managed to compete well enough to not only stay in business but actually show some patient growth. The credit for this was primarily due to the leadership talents of Mr. Frey coupled with a business strategy going back to the middle and late 1980s of actively competing for managed care contracts. The bad news was that managed care paid less to both doctors and hospitals. The other bad news was that, in 1997, we lost Mr. Frey.

This was not a minor issue. From the point he left and the time of the purchase of the Woodland facility in 1999, we were essentially leaderless but on autopilot using the structures and staff he'd put in place in those seven years. The issue that resulted in his leaving was twofold: he was offered a CEO position at a psychiatric hospital, at that time run by the for-profit company Charter, and he was not offered the COO position at Alexian Brothers Medical Center with the departure of Pat Paulson. In retrospect, this looks like one very bad decision by the corporate office, given that Mr. Frey is now the head of the entire Alexian Brothers Health System. But in 1997, he'd only worked in psychiatry and apparently hadn't had enough experience in the other areas of hospital operation. From the point of view of psychiatry, however, it eventually worked to our advantage. In 1999, he came back but in a somewhat different capacity as CEO of our "new" psychiatric hospital.

Between 1990 and 1999, the power of managed care to control hospital utilization grew exponentially. Office practice was affected to a lesser degree but still was substantially impacted. Whereas in the 1980s there was the threat of what managed care would/could do to hospital practice, in the 1990s there came the reality.

During the early and middle 1990s, the for-profit medical/surgical hospital companies had not done well in the Chicago area and by 1997 began to exit the Chicago market by selling off their assets here. One of these was Columbia Hoffman Estates Medical Center, which is still a very successful company in many parts of the country, but it couldn't make it here for whatever reason.

In the Alexian neighborhood they owned two hospitals, one of which was called Woodland, a psychiatric hospital, and the other a general hospital known as Columbia/HCA, located about three hundred yards to the west of the psychiatric hospital. That hospital had originally been built in the 1970s as Suburban Medical Center. It was an investor-owned facility later acquired by Humana (when it was a for-profit hospital company, before Humana decided that the real money is in being a health insurance company). It was later sold to for-profit Columbia before that company merged with Hospital Corporation of America (HCA) to become Columbia/HCA. Both hospitals were put up for sale in 1998.

As it turned out, a number of the remaining nonprofit hospitals entered into what amounted to a bidding war to obtain the general hospital. No one apparently was interested in the psychiatric hospital. It opened in 1990 and did well for about three, maybe four, years, but by 1998 it was losing about $250,000 a month, had diminishing admissions, and was physically deteriorating through lack of adequate maintenance. Psychiatry was on the ropes, and everyone knew it. The Alexian Brothers were willing to buy both hospitals, whereas the other bidders were only interested in the medical/surgical hospital. Their willingness to buy the psychiatric hospital was rumored to be a factor in Alexian's successful bid for the medical/surgical hospital. The Alexian Brothers also had a hospital in San Jose, California, and HCA was interested in an exchange of properties plus whatever the difference in cash value at the two sites. Whatever the arrangements, Woodland became the Alexian Brothers Behavioral Health Hospital in 1999. Mark Frey came back as CEO.

CHAPTER 13

MANAGED CARE TRIUMPHANT, OR "IT DEPENDS ON WHAT THE MEANING OF 'IS' IS"

I n April 1913, Sir William Osler[12] gave a series of lectures at Yale University, which in 1921 were published by Yale University Press as a volume titled The Evolution of Modern Medicine. In chapter 1 (lecture 1) on the origins of medicine, Osler says, "Medicine arose out of the primal sympathy of man with man; out of the desire to help those in sorrow, need and sickness ... The instinct of self-preservation, the longing to relieve a loved one, and above all the maternal passion-for such it is-gradually softening the hard race of man ..."

While "primal sympathy" may have been the origin of medicine and the

---

[12] Sir William Osler, often referred to as the "Father of Modern Medicine," was a physician who had a major impact on the profession primarily as a teacher. He was a Canadian who studied at various centers in Europe and, in 1888, became a founding professor of medicine at the new Johns Hopkins University Medical School. In 1892 (in the first four years of its existence there were no students at the medical school), he published a textbook, The Principles and Practice of Medicine. It was read worldwide and, in 1897, by one F. T. Gates, who was instrumental in advising John D. Rockefeller to fund the Rockefeller Institute of Medicine in New York. Osler is credited with starting the practice of presentation by students of patients they'd studied on hospital wards to service chiefs, which evolved into the clinic-pathologic conferences so common today. His compassion for people and respect for students made him famous.

original mission of the ancient Alexian Brothers, the insurance industry and the for-profit hospital world had no such obligation or history.

There's an axiom in the business world that goes, "Every problem is a potential opportunity." It is, of course, true. The cost of providing more and more care to more and more people is the problem. The opportunity came to be called managed care. Physicians and especially psychiatrists hated it but did little, in any organized or coherent way, to address the problems that gave it birth and nurturance.

After about 1992, managed care essentially dismantled the hospital practice of psychiatry as it was being practiced nationwide. Such was the case in medicine and surgery, as well, though much less pervasively. It didn't happen overnight, but it was progressive and inexorable. At Alexian Brothers, our willingness to work with managed care (known in those years as "The Great Satan") did not strike us as anything more than simple common sense. We realized there were excesses, and those excesses, as in any field, formed the bases of future problems for the profession and the patients we served. Moreover, it was a battle that could not be won. We treated inpatients, and, if we had any intention of continuing to do so, we simply had to find a way to make it work.

Despite the competition, we were able to maintain a reasonable patient census up through mid-1999, even though our relatively short lengths of stay were shortened further. At our major (primarily for-profit) competitor hospitals, the intrusions of managed care had a greatly magnified effect since they were highly dependent on very long lengths of stay, maximum prices for services, and the revenues those strategies generated. Initially these hospitals maintained the bizarre belief that they could somehow resist changes going on in the marketplace and behaved as though, somehow, it was all going to simply go away. It didn't.

Suing health plans was expensive, time-consuming, and (we believed) futile. We also knew there were widespread abuses that we felt negatively affected our competitiveness since we were unable or unwilling to compete on those terms.

We saw in the preceding chapter how the new Four Winds Hospital in Lamont, lacking an established referral base, was in foreclosure by July 1992 and being sued by stockholders in August of that same year. Although the hospital itself lasted until 2002, it was not a model of ethical operation, according to the lawsuits, not only by stockholders but ultimately by the federal government, as well. It's difficult to understand just what they were thinking. The others lasted a bit longer but ultimately came to a similar fate.

There were many players in the for-profit hospital business in 1992, and there still are, though now very few are psychiatric. A major psychiatric for-profit company was Psychiatric Institutes of America, which operated Linden Oaks Hospital in Naperville. As PIA began to unravel, Charter took over for a time until even they went under, and Linden Oaks, as of this writing, is fully a division of Edward Hospital in Naperville, a not-for-profit community hospital. Charter also operated Charter Barclay Hospital in Chicago at that time. Community Psychiatric Centers (CPC) operated Streamwood Hospital until CPC dissolved, although Streamwood Hospital continues under Universal Health, the nation's largest (and practically only) major for-profit psychiatric company, and survives locally by serving a very specialized population. In 1999, even the minor players were larger than Alexian Brothers.

From 1985 through 1987, I had the opportunity of serving as president-elect and president of the Illinois Psychiatric Society (IPS). Although I'd served on both ethics and insurance committees in previous years, two previous presidents, Drs. Patrick Staunton and Alex Spadoni, thought it was time for the local psychiatric society to get into the managed care debate and nominated me. They believed that there was no future in suing insurance companies. The office of IPS president allowed access to the debates about managed care in both Illinois and Washington, DC, where the American Psychiatric Association (APA) was headquartered. In 1986, managed care was a growing threat but still a minor player on the psychiatric stage. By 1999, it was in total control of at least the hospital branch of the profession and becoming very influential in office practice.

At the national level, both Dr. Greg Teas and I served on the APA's Managed Care Committee, where we witnessed venomous displays of anger and outrage but came away with the belief that, apart from the possible therapeutic value of cathartic displays of emotion, nothing useful could happen here. An association of competing interests and belief systems could not address the fundamental problems. The various irreconcilable factions dividing psychiatry at that time (some remaining in the present) rivaled those that wore down Renaissance Florence. We came to appreciate how difficult it is for a national organization to speak with one voice when members are divided with each group, using the threat of resignation if the organization takes a public position counter to their interests. Medical directors of some of the managed care companies (themselves members of the APA) would be invited to committee meetings, and a dialogue started, but these usually degenerated quickly into displays of anger and outrage. By 1999, "market forces" were in the ascendancy.

The factions (thusly characterized) most threatened by managed care were threefold. First, for purposes of discussion but very likely the smallest in actual numbers, were those intimate with the large hospital companies who were threatened by the potential for dramatically reduced lengths of stay, which would inevitably translate into growing numbers of empty beds. However, in the mid-1980s, large hospital companies were apparently telling doctors, stockholders, and themselves that further growth was indeed possible. In Chicago's northwest suburbs, four hospitals were on the drawing boards, and the Alexian Brothers department of psychiatry was wondering if it had a future.

Second were the psychiatrist members of the APA whose practices were more or less exclusively in the office. Many of these either were analysts or practiced one of the many varieties of psychotherapy practice in which long-term therapy was the rule. The twenty-outpatient-sessions-per-year benefit touted by many developing managed care companies was clearly a threat to their livelihood, as well as running counter to everything their years of training had been about. Managed care contracts usually contained specific exclusions for psychotherapy other than "crisis intervention," which they interpreted as treatment requiring less than twenty visits yearly. In practice, few actually got twenty visits, and the average was probably closer to six to eight visits annually. Before managed care, the average number of visits for psychiatric treatment across the nation was not very high. However, there were certain areas (urban versus rural, New York, Washington, Los Angeles, Chicago area north of interstate 80) and certain health plans (federal and state, IBM, GM, Champus) where utilization was reportedly very high.

A third group, comprising probably the largest group in terms of numbers, were perhaps not as outraged as were the first two but were indeed dismayed by the potential decrease in already-limited benefits for patients who needed them and the possible loss of autonomy in day-to-day practice that "managed" care implied. Long-term inpatient or outpatient treatment was not necessary for this group to earn a living. This group shared much with their medical colleagues outside psychiatry who themselves were uncertain of what the future would hold but were being told that "capitation" (caring for all the medical needs of a given population for a fixed monthly fee) was somehow in their future.

The issue of psychiatric insurance benefits has been historically difficult because of a lack of advocacy by those likely to need them. Because psychiatric conditions have been historically stigmatizing, it has been difficult to get patients to advocate for themselves. Insurance companies argued that no one wanted mental health coverage while then complaining that when included in health plans they were being overutilized.

In 1996, the opportunity to serve as representative from Illinois in the Assembly of the American Psychiatric Association from 1996 to 2002 presented itself. By this time the power of managed care to influence all aspects of psychiatric care was in full blossom. It was probably one of the most interesting decades in the history of American psychiatry, and, no, these changes were not paralleled in Europe or the rest of the world. This was strictly an American phenomenon.[13]

The debates, both locally and in Washington, DC, at the APA, were, as in 1986 to 1987, impassioned and took on a decidedly moralistic tone. Managed care was the "Great Satan" and the methods, well, satanic. The consequences would be disastrous for the mentally ill of the nation. Suicides would soar, and the ranks of the homeless would multiply. As it turned out, the ranks of the homeless appeared to increase, but this had little to do with the demise of the large hospital companies so dependent on private health insurance, which few of the homeless possessed.

Increases in homelessness among the mentally ill had more to do with decreasing public sector and community support services for chronic mental illness (services not usually supported by private insurance in any case), along with changes in mental health law that allowed many severely mentally ill to refuse needed treatment unless they tried to kill someone or tried (and failed, of course) to kill themselves. Dr. Darold Treffert, mental

---

[13] To say that cost is not an issue in the rest of the world is not what's implied in this statement. Working within a budget is part of health care everywhere. Managed care as encompassing and as intrusive as practiced here is unique to us.

health advocate and former head of the public mental health hospital system of the state of Wisconsin, referred to this liberalization of mental health law as allowing patients to "die with their rights on." Despite all the weeping and gnashing of teeth, economic forces were too compelling to be denied.

In looking at the managed care "revolution," it may be useful to start with what, in my opinion, was right about managed care in psychiatry particularly and in medicine generally. First, managed care was clearly a response to the perception that there was overuse and even outright abuse of health insurance, as it existed in the 1960s through the 1980s. This was absolutely the case in the psychiatric hospital world. While there were lots of complaints, certainly no professional organization was in any position to do anything since any action would invariably alienate someone. Therefore, unity of action couldn't happen. Managed care's mandate was to reduce utilization, and it did.

Second, in the absence of any kind of coherent national or even statewide health care system of any kind, doctors, patients, hospitals, pharmacies, and drug companies continued to behave in ways that served their own economic and emotional requirements. In medicine this financially exploitational element has been sarcastically referred to as a "wallet biopsy." One patient of mine was spending $95 per day on two pills of the antipsychotic drug olanzapine after failing to tolerate five or six others, including our most effective antipsychotic drug, clozapine. Luckily his family was capable of absorbing this kind of expense until olanzapine became generic, but few families are able to come up with $34,675 per year for one medication. The system needed some kind of oversight or management, which clearly still does not exist.

Third, it forced physicians and other professionals to look at what they were doing and why they were doing it. If someone is challenging what one does, one must offer some rational defense. The best defense is to base what one does on evidence rather than on quasi philosophical or political beliefs. Hysterectomy or tonsillectomy (and other surgical procedures) on demand and very long psychiatric hospital stays were no longer routinely available. This was not necessarily bad.

A national managed care company (or a national organization like Medicare) has access to data showing that professionals in different areas of the country or in different regions of the same state were treating the same patients in very different ways using different resources and at widely differing costs. Hysterectomies, vaginal versus cesarean deliveries, and a host of other surgical and diagnostic procedures varied considerably. In psychiatry, if a generalized anxiety disorder is being treated with weekly cognitive/behavioral psychotherapy in one town and with five-times-per-week psychoanalysis in another, it raises the question of why there were differences and whether the results of one form of treatment were truly superior to the other.

Without getting into a debate about which therapies were best, it opened the discussion about evidence-based treatment, which needed to occur. As with drugs, if one has a choice between treatments A and B, and A costs five or ten times more than B, it becomes incumbent upon the advocates of A to demonstrate superiority. In the case of drugs or medical devices, for example, that would mean going beyond buying lunches, dinners, or theater tickets for physicians to influence treatment decisions. The physician, in my opinion, has the obligation of "ethical stewardship" of resources and should avoid prescribing a drug that costs $800 per month if one comparable is available for $30, regardless of who's paying for it. Unfortunately, a few doctors saw profit in courting drug company favor and avoided using generic equivalents, always finding some questionable "quality" justification. As with everything else, advertising works, and only the most expensive drugs are advertised.

Managed care diminished greatly the control of child/adolescent admissions to hospitals and the lengths of stay while they were there, basically controlled by schools (in close cooperation with hospitals and some doctors) for many years. In fact, the most lucrative population for many private, freestanding psychiatric hospitals in the Chicago area was adolescents. Schools tended to favor longer stays, which suited the large hospital companies very well. Unlike younger children, adolescents tended to have older parents who were likely to be more stable financially and had better insurance.

After managed care, admission to a hospital came to be controlled more by the insurance company's "network" (and their reviewers) than by the schools. This did not seem inappropriate to many of us, since not all referral patterns in psychiatry (or in general medicine, for that matter) were appropriate (i.e., based strictly on patient need and cost). Cost can, should, and always will be a legitimate factor to consider in health care planning, whether we like it or not. Citizens of England and France get pretty good health care with better overall population health at considerably less cost.

There was a time when the timing of a child's reentry into school was dictated by when the school agreed to schedule a reentry staffing (a meeting in which the various interested parties in a particular case get together to discuss next steps). This could be many weeks, perhaps as long as a month. This was like asking a cab to wait outside for a month while the meter keeps running. When the meeting finally occurred, it could be a meeting of twenty-five or thirty people, when three or four would have been sufficient, which is what occurs today. Schools always had their reasons for needing twenty-five or thirty people to be at these meetings, which took so long to set up. That everyone thought they were doing best by the child was never in doubt, but today's more streamlined procedures seem to work just fine and at much less expense. Schools viewed medical/psychiatric financing in much the same way they looked at school financing. They viewed an insurance trust as not unlike a school budget. They saw these monies as "budgeted" and saw no rationale for "giving back" monies already in the budget.

Schools behaved as though they didn't understand that in the insurance world these costs are referred to as "losses," and insurance companies do not smile at the prospect of losses of any kind, whether generated by God or man. Schools didn't care that these losses were made up by yearly increases in premiums, which industry and government employers did not welcome and were determined to curtail. In a world where money was no object (in the "all we care about is quality" world), it could theoretically be tolerated, but those days were rapidly drawing to a close, and more objective definitions of quality were evolving.

Hospitals and doctors also reacted to the insurance company's loss mentality with some dismay. Here we thought we were doing good for patients, but when all is said and done, we're just another fire or hurricane where the insurance company is concerned, and the expectation from its board and stockholders is to find ways to get out of paying the bills or minimize their risk. One minimizes risk by not insuring sick people.

Managed care had, in my opinion, a positive effect in diminishing (though not entirely eliminating) questionable charges and services. As an occasional surveyor for the hospital licensing division of the Illinois

Department of Public Health during the 1980s, I became privy to a multitude of services and testing done with little notion of or concern for the usefulness or relevance of the results. Large psychiatric groups (that may have had ownership interests in the hospitals themselves) found creative ways of increasing the charges presented to insurers. Psychiatrists in some hospitals billed daily or almost daily but often, depending on the hospital, could find no order or even any note in the chart written personally by a psychiatrist. Orders were done almost entirely via phone. One psychologist presumably saw the patient in daily psychotherapy, while another in the same group did batteries of psychological testing routinely. In several hospitals a neurologist saw patients armed with his own staff of speech therapists, occupational therapists, and anyone else who could test someone for something and generate a bill.

If these tests were based on the specific needs of patients, there would have been no problem. Managed care organizations even today will authorize testing for specific justifications, but those seen were often routinely ordered on all patients, depending on their coverage, and one could almost never find any statement in the chart explaining just why they were necessary. In these cases the very existence of insurance resulted in the moral hazard that insurances were warning against. Today these abuses are less common but still occur occasionally. It would be the equivalent of a cardiologist performing cardiac catheterizations routinely on everyone regardless of indications, and, by the way, the cardiologist just happens to own the cath lab. In psychiatry, since these tests are not physically invasive and are of minimal physical danger to anyone, they were usually justified on the principles of "quality care," which is always the justification for more charges. Some doctors would present themselves as simply "obsessed with quality and thoroughness" (which unfortunately came with much larger charges). An added bonus was that the paper generated constituted de facto marketing documents when sent to schools but also raised the question of how much personal information a school required or had a right to.

Managed care may have even had some positive influence in the development of day hospital programs (DHP's) and intensive outpatient programs (IOP's) even if rather unintentionally. Early on, insurances were reluctant to fund day hospitals since patients stayed so long as inpatients. Day hospitals were seen as opportunities for perpetual treatment (some patients, when all is said and done, will need it, but the number is very small). When inpatient coverage began being cut and patients were sometimes still very obviously impaired, it became acceptable to fund day hospital programs as an alternative when patients remained ill but not obviously dangerous. These proved both less expensive as well as just as effective in many cases when patients were more stable and, while still quite ill, were in more of a subacute phase. Less expensive is good in that it allows a larger number of patients to have access to services that might otherwise be unavailable. Resources are no longer unlimited, if they ever were.

However, while managed care had some positives and reduced outright abuse of financial resources, it also had many negatives and abuses of its own. One glaring problem, then and now, is the absence of standards in reviewing the need for care. Some companies saw as their "Mandate of Heaven" the prevention of as much care (losses) as possible, whether medical or psychiatric. Some companies decided, rather self-servingly, that there were no justifiable reasons to hospitalize psychiatric patients short of actual suicide or homicide attempts, or psychoses so severe the patients required restraints or one-to-one coverage. Then they tried to write criteria to exclude even that if they could, which didn't work and invited backlash. Some insurers refused payment for the medical treatment of self-inflicted injuries. Therefore, a suicide attempt by overdose that required the patient to be placed on a ventilator, or a stab wound requiring surgical intervention, would often be disallowed under the "self-inflicted" exclusion. I never heard about denials of treatment for smokers or drinkers for medical problems resulting from these "self-inflicted" diseases.

As the large hospital companies were created to make lots of money quickly, the managed care companies and managed care divisions of insurance companies (admittedly created out of necessity) ultimately saw gold in the prevention of care, oftentimes by redefining the meaning of the word "necessary." This reminded us of President Clinton's lawyerly utterance, "It depends on what the meaning of 'is' is," during his impeachment hearings.

For example, many companies in the early days excluded what they called "chronic" psychiatric conditions, which were then deemed untreatable (by their own criteria) and thereby excluded from coverage. The premise here was that any attempt to treat an untreatable condition is a waste of resources (the insurance company's) and should not be attempted. No matter how ill the patient, such treatment can never be "medically necessary." Since there were still state mental hospital beds, the implication was that they could be referred there for care. State hospitals were psychiatric managed care's backup safety net.

Some cases were simply incredulous, like the one referred to the insurance committee. This was the case of a woman in her midthirties who was employed, had health insurance, developed an apparently psychotic illness, and ended up in an emergency room. Although very disorganized mentally, and recommended for admission by the ER doctor, she was coherent enough to deny that she was suicidal or homicidal. And she was neither. What that meant for insurance purposes was that she was not meeting that particular company's criteria for hospital admission. Still feeling she was too ill to send home for outpatient treatment, the ER doctor sent her to a nearby state hospital, which saw no justification for denying her. They agreed she was quite ill and, although not specifically suicidal or homicidal, seemed to show highly impaired judgment. Unfortunately for this patient, it was an uncommonly cold December in Chicago. Several days after admission, she was found frozen to death on the hospital grounds, having left the building somehow without a coat or shoes. She was never suicidal. Her death was accidental.

This case most likely became a legal problem for the state hospital in that this very ill woman was "allowed to leave" the closed setting of the hospital, and perhaps they were negligent. At that time also it was most unlikely the insurance company had any liability since all clinical decisions stayed with the medical personnel. The ER doctor could have kept her in the ER for twelve to twenty-four more hours, doing various levels of appeal, the company would argue. Besides, she was in a hospital. Citing lack of authorization, the insurance company was not going to let us look at any records. There was no further feedback on this, but maybe justice was ultimately served.

On the other hand, there are some serious conditions that sometimes warrant denial of certain types of care. Suppose some doctor tells his patients that he's found a wondrous new treatment for something like pancreatic cancer. He discovered it while traveling down the Amazon, where he ran into an Indian tribe that concocted a wondrous treatment from the venom of a rare snake that inhabits the jungle along the banks of the

Peruvian Amazon. Or maybe he's obtained it from a presumably respected American scientist who discovered a cancer cure in a laboratory somewhere while researching a cure for acne. If we read the published evidence on the treatment carefully, we find that the evidence base is comprised largely of testimonials from people presumably given up for dead by mainstream doctors who survived pancreatic cancer and now have no trace of it. Cure reports like these, based on testimonials, are common in otherwise hopeless diseases where some patients will pay anything for a chance at survival.

Unfortunately, this medication is given in a series of ten injections that cost $25,000 per injection (this particular Amazon serpent being very rare). Should Blue Cross, Medicare, or any insurance company pay for this? Certainly the disease is very real (if legitimately confirmed) and very deadly. There is no denying "necessity" on some level, but is the treatment likely to eliminate or even significantly slow down the progress of the cancer? In the absence of credible evidence, paying $375,000 for these injections is not warranted. Managed care has saved the insurer $375,000 in a patient highly unlikely to benefit. The patient's family will argue that they have nothing to lose by going through the treatment, and to them it seems cruel. In the absence of any credible evidence, spending $375,000 for this treatment is unwarranted. Too often the family finds the money, which is an expensive way to learn that the days of miracles have passed.

When looking at concept of psychiatric medical necessity, the same type of argument might apply but in a much more distorted way. Take the case of a psychotic person who does not respond to an antipsychotic medication within a week to ten days. What we saw with the advent of managed care is that this patient, even if only seventeen, might be characterized by the insurance reviewer as "chronic" and future psychiatric benefits disallowed. This was reprehensible, from my point of view, but at least there were state hospitals then. No longer.

To compare schizophrenia or an intense bipolar illness to something like gallstones (treatment of the former taking many months, and the latter just a few days) didn't make sense then or now. But even chronic psychiatric patients have better and worse days, weeks, and years and need treatment at certain times more than other times and are not perpetually in need of hospital care.

Diabetes is a chronic condition, especially when it starts in childhood or adolescence. Nevertheless, diabetics, especially certain younger patients, go into diabetic comas, have hypoglycemic episodes, and develop neuropathies or vision problems—lots of things for which it would be immoral, if not illegal, to refuse payment. For those with chronic medical conditions, the insurer's goal to this point in history has been to try very hard to avoid enrolling them. Refusing to enroll sick people over the last sixty years is the most obvious evidence that caring for the sick is not a specific mission of most health insurance companies or managed care organizations.

Patients with chronic medical conditions or parents or spouses of those with chronic conditions could in the past never leave one job for another, since getting health insurance for a preexisting condition was next to impossible. The Affordable Care Act (Obamacare) mandates otherwise but has been long in coming and (as of this writing) is being strongly lobbied for repeal. It is my belief (hopefully incorrect) that, should Obamacare not be repealed, insurance companies will find some way to circumvent the mandate or collect even more money to protect themselves against medical loss. In the final analysis, the insurer exists to prevent losses, not help sick people. In many cases a company will not participate, not so much because of the fear of actually losing money, but because they don't anticipate making enough money to satisfy investors. It is, in the end, a return-on-investment issue.

Early in the history of psychiatric managed care, organizations took the "chronic" loophole to extremes and narrowed the definition to include anyone the reviewer believed wasn't going to get well in seven or ten days (yes, we received denials after seven days in cases where the insurance's contractual obligation was only ten days, because the condition was "chronic"). After some public outcry, these criteria were relaxed somewhat, but even today we commonly see denials in which the terms "chronic" or "custodial" are used by managed care organizations to deny benefits. We have also noticed that since the passage of the Affordable Care Act, companies have become once again particularly ruthless. The reason here is that the Affordable Care Act mandates a degree of parity in psychiatric benefits, which means insurers can't simply exclude psychiatric and substance abuse benefits in health plans and can't impose limits they don't require for the treatment of other diseases. However, they can make it difficult to impossible to use these benefits.

Here's how it works: A patient is admitted to the hospital, let's say after a suicide attempt or possibly a psychotic episode. The indications for admission may be self-evident to everyone, even the insurance company. A treatment plan is implemented. Four or five days later, the care is "reviewed" again. If the patient happens to be better, then the case is reviewed again in two or three days and may be decertified at that point, because, in the case of the suicide attempt, the patient may answer no to the question "Are you suicidal?"

At this point the patient no longer meets that company's criteria for inpatient treatment. The criteria are written by the company to protect itself, so even the presence of suicidal thinking, after a serious suicide attempt, may disallow more hospital care. The criteria often read that the patient has to admit to a frank plan to kill himself to remain in the hospital since only thinking about it (the actual attempt may be only a few days ago) qualifies him for discharge to a day hospital program. Patients often say no to the suicide question, but how someone responds to such a question in a hospital and when out in the real world may be very different. Since this kind of situation does not lend itself to exact predictions, it becomes a matter of opinion and clinical intuition. I have one opinion since I see the patient daily. The reviewer, however, who's never seen the patient, has another. Sometimes this flies in the face of common sense, and it becomes difficult or impossible to explain to a frightened family why their insurance will no longer certify when neither the doctor nor the family believes the patient is ready for discharge. If the family complains, they're always told that the attending physician makes the final decision, which is technically true since the insurance company doesn't (it claims) make "clinical" decisions, only financial ones. Of course, the financial decisions are based on what? Clinical data, of course. Why do we have to give clinical data daily anyway?(It depends on what the definition of "is" is.) In situations like this, which occur daily, we're not trying to decide if we'll keep the patient for three or four months. We're arguing about three or four days.

The company will argue that (here's where it gets interesting) clinical decision-making is not their charge. It's the doctor's role, and all liability stays with the person making the clinical decisions. Their obligation is simply to pay for the care as their criteria dictate, and their criteria do not allow payment beyond a certain date, after which payment becomes the obligation of the patient. Of course, there are elaborate appeal processes that have to be done within certain time frames, always with reviewers working with the same criteria. These appeals may take some time, and if the patient stays in the hospital, and we don't win the appeal, then the patient and/or the hospital takes the hit. The fact that the insurance company's position about the clinical decision-making process is belied by the fact that they will often demand that certain medications be prescribed, or changed, or increased based on their clinical opinions, sometimes lab tests demanded, with days disallowed if one doesn't comply. The goal here is for the insurance company to maintain maximum control over treatment and length of stay while making it clear that all liability for the welfare of patients remains squarely on the shoulders of the physician and hospital. Our moral and legal obligation is to act in the best interest of the patient regardless of consequences. Insurance companies' obligations are contractual, and their adherence to their internally written criteria is all they need to worry about. All criteria are based on whether or not patients say they're suicidal or homicidal at the moment of review. If they're in a safe environment, of course they won't necessarily be consumed by suicidal urges, but whether they're ready to leave the sheltered environment of the hospital is another matter.

Another example is a twenty-two-year-old woman with a history of treatment for depression. She attempts suicide by overdosing on twelve extra-strength Tylenol tablets after a breakup with a boyfriend. This is a first attempt that anyone knows about. She had a blood alcohol level of 0.06 (below the legal limit of 0.08). She's treated at a local hospital emergency room where those who evaluate her feel that she remains emotionally unstable (still just as upset as she was before overdose) and needs psychiatric hospitalization. The hospital closed its psychiatric service last year, as it was too unprofitable, so they call Alexian Brothers, where there is an available bed. The insurance company disagrees with the recommendation for hospitalization and will take one of two positions. They could decide that the patient is not in need of hospitalization, and they will not certify her but will review her case the following day. If we can convince them that she really is "imminently dangerous" (which means she will definitely kill herself today if discharged today), they may certify something, days to be determined. Otherwise, they will certify one day, but within twenty-four hours we must prove to their satisfaction that she is still dangerous and requires more time.

From the insurance perspective, there are many signs of ambivalence on the patient's part about death. For instance, the bottle had thirty-six tablets, but she only took twelve. It was done within less than forty-eight hours of the breakup so perhaps can be considered impulsive without much premeditation. She told her boyfriend what she'd done, so he called an ambulance. She did not choose death by hanging or shooting, which would have been more effective. Maybe she didn't really want to die. These are issues that we need to look at, but in the final analysis our obligation is not to prevent insurance losses but to do what's in the best interest of someone who has now become our patient. In a case like this one, the insurance company has already made a decision. If our decision concurs with theirs, then it's not a problem. If it differs—if we believe the patient to be still unstable while even sober—instead of focusing on what the treatment plan needs to be, we now have to spend time debating criteria. The problem is that one party in this debate has moral and legal obligations, and the other has contractual obligations.

There is also a significant difference between not being suicidal in a hospital environment and not being suicidal outside of a hospital. This is not a matter of all or nothing, like being pregnant or not. In the real world, emotions change rapidly depending on a multitude of variables. The high-risk time for completed suicides is shortly after being discharged from a hospital. Even patients who are honest in their reports underestimate the crush of real-life experience upon discharge from a hospital. In cases like these, the opinion of the psychiatrist means a great deal while, at the same time, very little. There are multiple appeals available, basically to protect the managed care company, so in the event the patient kills herself, they can say the error here was entirely mine since the psychiatrist makes the clinical decisions and they only make financial decisions. The insurance company, by its criteria, can predict what the patient will and will not do. The average "pretty good" doctor cannot. It depends on what the definition of "is" is.

An attending psychiatrist can expect to spend lots of time on this case on the day of admission, or on subsequent days, depending on whether or not he agrees with the insurer. The secret goal here is to frustrate the psychiatrist into getting the patient out as soon as possible and not act in the patient's best interest. Dr. Spadoni (chapter 1) reports that psychiatrists are abandoning hospital practice. One wonders why.

In a recently published study of the number of hours spent weekly by US physicians in administrative work, psychiatry beat out all other specialties at 9.6 hours or 20.3 percent of all hours worked (Woolhandler and Himmelstein 2014). The average for all physicians was 8.7 hours or 16.6 percent.

In the case of a frankly psychotic person admitted to a hospital, the same process works in the same way. If the person is better in five or seven days, then fine. If the person is not, then we go to more frequent reviews. Since the advent of Thorazine and the rest of the antipsychotics, it generally takes much less hospital time to show some improvement in psychosis, but the hard reality is that not everyone is equally responsive in the hoped-for time frames. If the patient does not respond within five to ten days, not only do we stand to get more frequent reviews, but also we now notice that certain words begin to creep into the conversation—words like "chronic" and "custodial," which are the secret words for "not included in our contractual obligation." The logic here is that if the patient does not respond quickly to a given treatment, then the insurance company has to begin to position itself in defense of losses. If we implement one treatment plan and are not successful within seven or eight days, then we have to change it quickly or run the risk of having the patient labeled "chronic" and the treatment "custodial." If that plan fails, then more days have elapsed, the words "chronic" and "custodial" are mentioned more and more, and it's clear where this conversation is going. Even when a patient is responsive to a treatment plan, it's a long way from a patient going from complete confusion and a belief that he's been marked for death by malevolent forces, to an ability to walk out the door and drive a car (to outpatient treatment) or function in a job or classroom. Even in responsive patients, the time between discharge and return to premorbid functional levels may vary from weeks to months to sometimes never. Relapse is frequent, because patients often look better to clinicians and insurers than they really are in the structured and generally supportive environment of a hospital.

Even today utilization standards vary greatly from company to company. Practitioners like myself see patients on a daily basis having coverage by two insurance companies (e.g., parents divorced, but the child, including those of college age and older, is covered by the health plans of both parents). One company will see the treatment as justified, and the other may not—so much for the myth of standardization, even in 2018. We experience on a daily basis insurance denials that are based simply on length of stay and no other criteria. If the patient is better, they'll demand discharge based on lack of need. If the patient is not better, they'll demand discharge based on lack of capacity to improve. All this in seven or eight days! From an insurance perspective, if a patient leaves a hospital and doesn't die, success has been achieved regardless of clinical condition.

The days when treatment was a private issue between doctor and patient are over forever in the United States. The insurance company has everything to say about every aspect of a patient's care, except when something goes wrong. The pendulum has now swung in the other direction, especially in psychiatry. That's why available psychiatric beds are decreasing and emergency rooms are filling up (chapter 1).

That said, we also see situations where these pressures I've written about do not occur. Why in one case we're given latitude to do what we think best (within reason) and in others every day is a struggle is unclear, but somehow there is some "invisible hand" operating somewhere in the private health insurance world. Whether this invisible influence comes from employers who are self-insured and only use insurers as "fiscal intermediaries" who process claims but do not pay them or through some other influence is not readily apparent. My suspicion is that, as a percentage of total medical costs, psychiatric care is not out of line, and some plans and/or employers do not seem inclined to squeeze their enrollees.

Instituted as a strategy to control cost, the greatest problem with managed care today is its incredible cost. Perhaps it was a necessary evil given the overutilization and financial exploitation, which no doubt did occur. However, today we have hordes of personnel at hundreds of insurers processing information, duplicating work, with armies of review personnel both at hospitals and insurers and most of it having little to do with caring for patients. Overhead plus profit has varied over the years, but 25 percent of the entire insurance premium has been common for most of the last twenty-five years, with some reports of insurers getting away with spending less than 50 percent of premiums for actual care. Rules under the Affordable Care Act try to increase the percentage of premiums devoted to taking care of the sick, but hopefully you will forgive me if I seem unduly skeptical. The influence of the insurance industry is so powerful and pervasive that with the combination of creative accounting and political clout, only the patients and providers are likely to lose.

While we're laying off nurses and other hospital staff who work directly with patients, insurers and hospitals spend millions weekly on advertising budgets. Up to and including the present, insurers spend heavily to attract and keep the healthiest populations and, as we've seen in managed Medicare in Illinois, try to disenroll sick patients or, if that's not possible, drop the plans entirely. Some plans will enroll Medicare patients on a county-by-county basis, depending on whether or not there's real money to be made.

Wanting to make money is not immoral. I'm sure the people who run health insurance companies are as good and moral a group of individuals as there are in the medical and other professions. The problems are in the incentives. But business is business, and when the bell rings, the name of the game is win, and excuses are not sympathetically received. The fact here is that health care is not the mission of insurance. The people are good, but the incentives are perverse for companies and for doctors, as well.

Medicare and, to a lesser extent, Medicaid began in 1966 with one mission only: to care for sick people. There is no better health insurance than Medicare. It enrolls the oldest and sickest populations and manages to get by with administrative expenses of about 3 percent. When enrolling in managed Medicare plans, many seniors don't really understand that they no longer have Medicare. The juxtaposition of the word "managed" with the word "Medicare" is mistakenly interpreted by aging seniors (I'm included in the "aging seniors" population) as their having some form of Medicare but with lower drug costs. If they should actually get sick, especially psychiatrically, reality comes a-calling. When the patient learns the truth and reenrolls in "real" Medicare at the next opportunity, they're doing exactly as hoped for. Insurance companies want the sick to disenroll sooner than later. Sick folks are not profitable.

The reason that there are incessant advertisements for automobile insurance everywhere is that each company is trying to attract the other company's lowest-risk drivers and divest themselves of the higher-risk drivers. Perhaps one can argue that driving is a matter of personal responsibility. All accidents require that someone be at fault so that there's someone to sue. In most accidents, someone probably is to blame, though sometimes both parties share blame. But with sickness we usually don't need to find who's to blame before we offer treatment, even though there may be plenty blame to go around. The patient smoked too much or drank too much or ate too much or had unprotected sex, but since one can't sue the patient (and the tobacco companies have paid out their billions, so now we can't say we never realized that smoking was bad for us), one is still ethically obligated to treat. Besides, even the nonsmokers and the teetotalers and the svelte will get something if they live long enough. Everyone is going to need medical care at some point.

Taking care of healthy people is where the money is (for insurers), and taking care of sick people loses money in much the same way that property insurers lose money in a hurricane. Although a hurricane is an intermittent event, sickness is ongoing and inexorable. The older the population gets, the greater the frequency of sickness. We have no cure for aging, and we are not likely to find one in the foreseeable future.

In the process of setting up health care exchanges at the state level, I noted a newspaper article recently citing the fact that a major for-profit insurance company had elected to not participate. Good moneymaker? Participate. Not profitable? Do not participate. The name of the game is "don't insure anyone we think might get sick if we can help it." Try having diabetes or any serious chronic condition in the past sixty years (including depression or any form of mental illness), and before the recent government mandated changes in health law, try to find health insurance. Having been in practice for many years, it's relatively common for me to see patients who I'd seen when they were teenagers come to see me ten or twenty years later to ask me if there's anything I could do for them since they'd been turned down for health or life insurance, despite many years of relatively healthy functioning. The odds are always in favor of the insurance company, much like the "house" at a gambling casino.

So we're evolving a system wherein the really sick elderly go on regular Medicare, the "active seniors" go on managed Medicare, and the lower quartiles of the population go on Medicaid (even more under the Affordable Care Act). So why do the insurers exist? The disquieting reality is that health insurers exist to make as much money as they can, taking care of the healthiest segment of the population. Yes, insured children get diabetes and leukemia and other bad things, but as a rule, they're healthy. Most pediatric care is "well care," as it should be.

Insurance companies don't like psychiatric benefits, because a majority of the seriously mentally ill become ill at relatively younger ages. A common time of onset of schizophrenia is eighteen to twenty-four and bipolar illnesses fourteen to thirty-five. In the health insurance world it is always more profitable to enroll the relatively young. Psychiatric illness in this age group lowers the profitability equation. Up to now, this has been the name of the game.

One of the Obamacare repeal-and-replace options under discussion as this is being written has to do with eliminating the parity requirement of Obamacare and going back to allowing companies to eliminate or minimize psychiatric and substance abuse benefits along with the requirement that young people buy health insurance. These options assume that people can know if they'll become sick or need treatment even though serious illnesses usually occur unpredictably or accidentally or are preexisting. However, insurance companies want to enroll healthy people, and giving young adults the option of enrollment means only the sick will sign up, with dramatic increases in premiums.

Perhaps preventing too much care (the only reason for managed care's invention) justified profits for the industry in the past. Americans spend more money for medical care, per capita, even with managed care, than any other developed nation in the world. Even with the Affordable Care Act, we still have a large percentage of the population without coverage. If we try to understand where the money goes (comparing the United States to other developed economies), we spend a whole lot more on drugs and administration than other countries and get back essentially nothing for the extra expense. The journal Health Affairs (September 2014) reported on hospital administrative costs in the United States and other countries (Himmelstein 2014). In the United States, 25.3 percent of hospital budgets go for administration compared to 12 percent in Canada and Scotland, and about 15 percent in France and Germany. On a per capita basis, the United States spends $667, Canada $158, Scotland $164, and England $225. The study found no evidence that the high US costs translated into better care or yielded any other benefits.

The United States ranks low on multiple measures of "quality" in the developed world. Do you feel the United States has "the best health care in the world"? For some of us "yes," but for many, if not most, of us, "no." Do we really believe that the citizens of France, England, Germany, or Canada get inferior care? If one believes in national health statistics, they seem to be doing pretty well, and they cover psychiatric conditions, as well, with much less angst.

The United States has no health care "system." We have many systems that are everywhere in competition with each other, but the competition is for the healthy and wealthy, while those who are truly sick or old (as a population) are paid for by the taxpayers or by the providers. For producing quality automobiles, competition works pretty well. For producing healthy citizens, because of perverse incentives, it doesn't seem to be working. What does a nonsystem look like? Each entity in a nonsystem works to its greatest financial advantage. A private health insurance company has no plan for reducing morbidity and mortality associated with common diseases, infant mortality, or sexually transmitted diseases, or otherwise improving the health of citizens. It may have a call-in service staffed by nurses, and it may want to have the better treatment organizations in its network. But in the end, its only concern is the people who pay its premiums, and if they don't make the profits they project, they either raise the rates or drop the coverage. Every private entity does that. Providers are no different. Some areas have loads of providers (doctors and hospitals, profit and nonprofit), and some areas have very few. This distribution is not based on population. This is what a nonsystem looks like. Insurance organizations justify their existence by preventing as much care as possible and lobby strongly against any kind of coherent system. What kind of system is it where almost no one pays the same price for a given service?

The lack of a system makes everything more expensive. Millions of dollars are spent weekly nationwide in advertising insurance plans. One insurance company has its own full-time cable channel that does nothing but advertise itself 24-7. When I was home nursing a broken bone, I watched hundreds of TV advertisements for various health care organizations. These must be costing millions. Pharmaceutical companies are now allowed direct-to-the-public advertising, ostensibly to "educate the public" about their options. If that was truly the case, why are only the most expensive drugs advertised? When was the last time anyone saw an advertisement for a generic drug? If the goal is educating the public, why not advertise the generic option? Drug advertising simply allows the companies to influence patient choices toward the most expensive options, and it works very well. Patients choose the more expensive drugs because they're advertised despite the availability of cheaper, equivalent options in most cases. Since the passage of the Affordable Care Act, generic drug shortages have developed, and 100 to 500-plus percent increases in drug costs are happening. Competition is lowering costs? If you believe that, you need a good psychiatrist.

Take Ford or Toyota, for example. If they ran their operations like they were health care organizations, and automobiles were paid for by health insurance, the Ford Focus, costing about $20,000, would cost $40,000. Why? Imagine a manufacturing operation where the cost of parts, labor, transportation, and availability vary dramatically on a day-to-day basis. This is US health care.

Automobile development and production are about as systems-oriented as they can be. If they don't control both cost and quality, eventually the advertising agency they hired won't be able to cover up all the flaws, and the company will inevitably go out of business (or have to get rescued by the taxpayers). Our nonsystem is constantly rescued by taxpayers who are paying at least 52 percent of the total health outlay (Himmelstein, Woolhand, and Hellander 2001). There are no "free market" miracles in serving the unprofitable. I can choose to buy a Ford or a Toyota or not. I cannot choose to remain well. And if I go to a hospital, they have a legal and moral obligation to treat me. Ford or Toyota dealers do not have a legal or moral obligation to give me a car.

Competition in most industries generally results in improved quality at lower cost. In health care, insurance companies do not develop newer treatments, and in no way are they involved in medical research other than cost equations. The federal government and private foundations support research. Pharmaceutical and device companies support research. The federal government (at least traditionally) has supported education and training, as have universities and hospitals. Unlike Ford or Toyota, competition between insurance companies does not result in better health. Health insurance companies may facilitate or retard specific treatments, drugs, or devices by virtue of what they agree to pay for, but they generally do not contribute to their development. Since the federal government is intimately involved in the evaluation of new products and treatments through the FDA and other regulatory agencies, insurance companies can access government data at no cost to themselves to decide what they will and will not pay for.

Insurance companies are immune from many government-mandated services with which hospitals and doctors are expected to comply. Yes, government (state or federal) may mandate coverage for psychiatric, substance abuse, or preventive gynecology services of some kind, but insurance companies simply charge more to cover their "risk." The same does not apply to hospitals and doctors. There are no billing codes for doing time-consuming reviews or appeals. Why is that?

Some Americans complain that "we" don't want a government takeover of health care. What those who say that really mean is that we don't want a government takeover of profitable health care, but we have no objection to the government funding of unprofitable health care. I'm puzzled by complaints about the government coming "between you and your doctor," when most insurers are very much in between you and your doctor and at considerable expense. As a practicing physician, I spend lots of time on the phone reporting or arguing with reviewers, but not when I'm lucky enough to have a Medicare patient. Even public aid, although reviewed, is more reasonable and less contentious. It may have something to do with mission (i.e., the reasons they exist).

Those TV ads during the debates on Obamacare showing that your plumber doesn't want a government "takeover" were paid for by the insurance companies who don't want a government "takeover" but still want to pick and choose just who they will or will not insure and at what cost. The modern myth is that medical decisions are a doctor/patient prerogative. The reality is that the insurance company decides regardless of what the patient or doctor wants. The insurance companies will claim that these decisions are based on some kind of scientifically derived criteria but, in fact, are usually based on the opinions of individual reviewers with no more clinical experience than the doctor they're arguing with and usually much less. All these insurance people need to be paid, and paid rather well, so much of the "savings" goes into administrative expenses.

Medicare has plenty of rules and regulations, but they tend to be uniform and do not require day-to-day begging by the physician and/or patient. Medicare has a particularly unpleasant program of after-the-fact payback if they find, in their after-the-fact review of cases, that days or admissions were not warranted. However onerous this practice, it isn't done while the patient is in the hospital, and it doesn't involve frantic and time-consuming phone calls. The rules may seem arbitrary, but we at least know what they are. Medicare is sensitive to public opinion, because patients can't be disenrolled. Private insurance is incentivized to encourage sick patients to find some other insurance plan if patients don't like them since they win when someone who's sick goes to a competitor.

The US Supreme Court recently ruled that it is not unconstitutional to require someone to buy health insurance. Some argued (rather emotionally) that requiring insurance is a violation of our American right to choose. Of course, that right to choose does not extend to a hospital having a right to choose not to treat an uninsured patient if insurance is available but not chosen by the patient.

In Illinois we have a law requiring, with little public outcry, licensed drivers to buy auto liability insurance, which graciously provides the legal profession the incentive to sue those involved in auto accidents. The Illinois legislature, famous for their diligence in financial matters, evidently wanted to make sure that all the lawyers get paid (the plaintiff's and the defendant's), which perhaps wouldn't always happen if car drivers had the right to choose. The hospitals and doctors who treat the injured from the same accidents are okay to be on their own and hope for public aid to cover 15 cents on the dollar since it would be unthinkable for the twenty-five-year-old who crashed his motorcycle into a light pole (but refused to get health insurance because then he couldn't afford the motorcycle) to go untreated. The mandatory auto insurance law did not require the Supreme Court's intervention, but the medical insurance law did. Why was that?

Health care is not a commodity that one can take or not take, as one can buy or not buy a car. In this country one traditionally has needed to be well to get health insurance, and it has been virtually impossible to get if one is sick. Both hospitals and doctors have legal and ethical obligations to treat the sick. Only insurance companies have no obligations toward anyone except their selected enrollees yet are the most powerful and most protected entities in health care.

Even with Obamacare, the young and presumably healthy are not signing up in the numbers needed. Trump is advocating for Obamacare repeal, therefore creating uncertainty (deliberately) in the insurance market.

Therefore, the cost for those who sign up will be much higher than originally anticipated since many of those who sign up will be those who've been denied in the past because of preexisting conditions. What we know for sure is that the insurers will not lose money and will do whatever they need to do to prevent as much care as possible, even while increasing rates as much as they want, so the end result will be at least twenty-five million uninsured even without Obamacare repeal. That is a lot of uninsured.

If cost is the issue, and we know it is, then the present nonsystem needs to be junked. For what Americans spend each year on health care, we (collectively) should have better. There is no way we'll ever again see the kind of unregulated access to care (for the well insured) that we saw in the 1960s and 1970s. Some kind of utilization and cost control is inevitable and necessary, but daily harassment of physicians is counterproductive, saves little money overall, and makes the practice of medicine extremely frustrating.

Step one is to eliminate employer-based health insurance. Step two is to get rid of the current insurance company role and establish a single-payer system so everyone has health insurance, we all play by the same rules, and the money we spend on health care goes to health care and not everywhere else. Those who oppose the single-payer system will shock everyone with ads about the cost to taxpayers. What they won't say is that by deducting the amounts already paid to private insurance companies, what's left will be the real cost, which will be less than we already pay. Insurance companies will still have a role, if they want, in the way they currently function as fiscal intermediaries in Medicare. The current system is not working, because it is, in fact, not a system. The Health Affairs article referred to above estimates that hospital overhead could be reduced by $150 billion annually by instituting a single-payer system (Himmelstein). A single-payer system would not eliminate competition between hospitals that would continue to be rewarded financially by more efficient and safer operations. As a physician it's clear that billing one entity with uniform rules is infinitely cheaper than billing fifty entities all with different forms and policies. As former Illinois Senator Everett McKinley Dirksen once remarked, "a billion here, a billion there, pretty soon we're talking real money."

CHAPTER 14

THE TROUBLE WITH PSYCHIATRY

First Thesis: Our knowledge is vast and impressive. We know not only
innumerable details and facts of practical significance, but also many
theories and explanations which give us an astonishing intellectual insight
into dead and living objects, including ourselves, and human societies.

Second Thesis: Our ignorance is boundless and overwhelming. Every
new bit of knowledge we acquire serves to open our eyes further
to the vastness of our ignorance. Both of these theses are true.

—Karl R. Popper, 1963

Mind is a series of operations carried out by the brain,
much as walking is a set of operations carried out by
the legs, except dramatically more complex.

—Eric Kandel, 2006

Mind–Body Dualism

In the twenty-first century, there are still plenty of troubles with
psychiatry. For some of us it is, in some perverse way, part of the attraction.
To begin with, psychiatric problems have for millennia been seen more as
social or moral than medical, and punishment seems to have been regarded
as an appropriate intervention. Unfortunately, this was more often than
not unsuccessful at getting these presumed sinners to change their ways
of thinking and behaving. There were other, more compassionate religious

views, which considered the mentally ill as part of God's creation, and as difficult as they were to understand or tolerate, they deserved compassionate care and treatment. On the other hand, some psychiatric patients have impressed their communities in ways that allowed them to appear especially "spiritual" and have at times been accepted as prophets with sometimes bizarre, occasionally deadly, consequences.

In more modern times, the medical nature of psychiatric conditions seems to be more accepted than in the past, but the prospect of having a disordered mind is still more concerning for many than having a disordered liver or even a disordered heart, although the latter can mean instant death at any moment, while a disordered mind usually does not. After all, your mind is you! Your heart can be replaced and is therefore not you! Nevertheless, to many patients, death can be a very attractive alternative to unremitting suffering and unending misery, which is the experience of many who experience serious and horrifying mental symptoms.

Notice use of the term "mind" as opposed to "brain" in this context. The use of these two different words for what may be the same thing has very different implications. The brain is a tangible thing, an organ with specific shape and structure made up of very specific types of tissue, which can be examined grossly and microscopically or imaged much like a heart or a kidney can be imaged. We have a rather good idea about what a heart or a kidney does, but when it comes to the creation of mind, how does the brain do it? How do we measure it? Mind is different ... or is it?

We can probably all agree that without a brain, there is no mind. But is it proper to say that a disorder of the mind necessarily involves a disorder of the brain? As of this writing, a majority of psychiatrists (and if not a majority, at least a significant minority of psychologists) would agree that a disordered mind is a manifestation of a disordered brain, at least in the more severe varieties. This was not the case as recently as the 1970s and 1980s, when Dr. Szasz's writings were so well received, and as chapter 10's reference to Dr. Eric Kandel's experience reports. Nor is this a concept universally accepted by all mental health professions even today.

As you may recall, Kandel was interested in psychoanalysis (the operation of the mind) at the time he trained at Massachusetts Mental Health but dismayed at how thoroughly the mind had become dissociated from the brain. He felt strongly that the various emotional phenomena observable in clinical psychiatry and in psychoanalysis (delusions, hallucinations, depression, repression, denial, anxiety, obsessions, and constructs like the ego, id, and superego) had some correlate or mechanism in the brain. These he felt could at some point be studied and ultimately yield knowledge worthy of the effort. As far as the faculty at Harvard (Massachusetts Mental Health) was concerned, Kandel's was a minority opinion.

The mind/brain dichotomy introduced a Cartesian dualism (body versus soul) into psychiatry with which no other medical specialty has had to deal. René Descartes was a seventeenth-century French mathematician and philosopher who proposed that humankind has a dual nature: the body, which is material in nature and includes the brain; and the soul, which is immaterial and eternal. This duality includes two types of substances: the res externa flowing through the nerves and activating muscles with animal spirits, and the res cogitans, which is only found in humans and is nonphysical.

Since we are completely in the dark about how the physical brain creates the psychological phenomena of the conscious mind, psychiatry has spoken two "languages" for some time and is likely to continue in that mode for a while. For better or worse, until a unifying language develops, psychiatrists must deal with the phenomena of mind and brain simultaneously and at the same time separately.

In general medicine and surgery, there are ongoing issues of legitimate competition related to overlap in training. For example, is the spine the province of the neurosurgeon or the orthopedist? For implanting cardiac devises, where does the skill of the cardiologist end and the cardiovascular surgeon begin? To the extent that what constitutes mind is so vast and includes such varied entities as religion and philosophy, politics and social theory, it makes sense for psychiatrists to limit psychiatry's scope to the more obvious areas that we call mental illness and leave philosophy to the philosophers and religion to the clergy. For many psychiatrists, this is still very difficult to accept, but it is not as bad as it once was. There is no reason to believe that the religious and philosophical views held by psychiatrists are any more insightful or valid than those held by other medical or surgical practitioners, or anyone else for that matter. We may have great interest but generally no special expertise in these matters.

However, since many psychiatrists have seemed more interested in metaphysics and philosophy, the result has been to make medical treatment in psychiatry look particularly onerous. Certainly not every medical treatment in psychiatry has been useful and safe. In chapter 6 we discussed psychosurgery, which was clearly overused and underevaluated (though with exceptions that I reviewed). Based on the knowledge of the time, not every case was inappropriate or inevitably harmful. I've tried in this monograph to deliberately look at psychiatry in the context of general medicine and surgery for a reason.

If we look at the many years of radical procedures in cancer treatment (e.g., radical mastectomies) only to learn that they were disfiguring while at the same time ineffective (compared to less radical procedures), we have not condemned them in the same way. Clearly physicians were doing what they sincerely believed was in the patients' best interest and were trying to save their lives. For most of my years in medicine, estrogen replacement was considered a rational practice based on what appeared to be common sense. Estrogen appeared to protect women from many of the disease states that afflicted aging men. So when oral estrogen became available, it seemed to be a good thing until, after many years of careful follow-up, it turned out otherwise. Practice rather abruptly changed when the data became available, but it was not a moral but a scientific issue. I'm sure there were lawsuits—there always are—but I didn't see medicine demonized for the practice. It seemed like common sense sixty-five years ago, and it took careful study over many years to find the truth. My own mother had her ovaries removed in the 1940s, was on estrogen replacement for over fifty years, thought she was living more comfortably, and lived to eighty-five. Not every woman had a bad outcome, which was why it took so long to gather useful data.

In the medical/surgical world, we make mistakes. In psychiatry, we commit sins.

The Patients

Another trouble with psychiatry in years past has been the patients. The actual patient population can be quite varied and range from the very psychotic who don't want to be anyone's patient willingly, to the high functioning who experience a wide variety of psychiatric symptoms but who actively seek out treatment. The common denominator has been an unwillingness to acknowledge themselves as members of the psychiatric patient population. This is why confidentiality has been an obsession in the profession long before HIPAA laws were passed for medicine in general. This is the problem of stigma and, almost by definition, defines a moral dimension. As psychiatrists (and for psychiatry), what this has meant is that we (and the patients we see) are spoken about in the media and in literature and the arts, but rarely favorably except during certain brief eras. If society as a whole thinks poorly of the patient population, then they're unlikely to think well of those who treat them. For some, the function of psychiatry is to keep the insane from preying on the sane, although the reverse is more often the case.

Over the years, speaking practically, stigma has meant that diagnosing anyone with anything psychiatric has been tantamount to calling them "crazy," and that has never been a good thing. The word "crazy" serves several functions: On the one hand, it is most often used colloquially in daily conversation to impugn the behavior and opinions of those who disagree with us ("You're crazy if you think the Bears are going to win the division."). It is also used colloquially to refer to people who may be psychotic or severely depressed but harkens back to the culture's earlier view of mental illness as a moral rather than a medical problem. "Psychotic" is medically correct but can also be used as an insult. Saying a person has pneumonia or cancer is not generally considered an insult, with exception perhaps for some sexually transmitted diseases.

Psychiatrists have seen this typically, over the years, on consultations requested in general medical/surgical hospitals, though things are changing in recent years. A good example is a patient who presents in a hospital emergency room with intense chest pain and discomfort, along with difficulty breathing. The possibility of a myocardial infarction (heart attack) certainly needs to be ruled out. This is a condition that can kill quickly and requires aggressive treatment in a timely fashion. To be worked up and then be told that the condition is not going to be fatal or damaging to heart tissue would normally be welcomed by someone who came into the ER thinking this day might be his last. And yet it appears that some patients seem rather disappointed if a diagnosis of an anxiety disorder is made and psychiatric consultation suggested. The patient has come to the hospital for help and instead may see the diagnosis and the consultation request as an insult ("This doctor thinks I'm crazy.").

For what should be great news, the feeling is often one of humiliation and embarrassment, as if the chest pain, shortness of breath, and heart rate of 145 was not real. This can lead to the patient's request for another doctor or another hospital, so doctors historically have made referrals to psychiatry with understandable reluctance. While things have changed over the past forty years, many patients still feel stigmatized by the hint of any psychiatric diagnosis and seem willing to undergo sometimes harrowing and dangerous diagnostic procedures to look for obscure and rare conditions to prove that they're not "crazy."

The problem of stigma raises issues on two levels. As illustrated above, if being a psychiatric patient is a potential source of humiliation and shame, then even those who willingly come for treatment are not going to admit to having been treated, and the rest will do everything they can think of to avoid it. The other is if there are no patients lobbying for better treatment or better financing of treatment, then the insurance industry has argued traditionally against inclusion of psychiatric benefits because "nobody wants it."

Without active lobbying, the states find public mental health budgets easy to cut, and even the willing get nothing. The result has for years been major decreases in public and private psychiatric bed capacity and the two-tiered payment system in private health insurance whereby psychiatric services are paid to a lesser degree (100 percent if "medical" and 50 percent if psychiatric; no limits on hospital days and office visits for "medical" and severe limits on psychiatric hospital days and office visits). This practice is reminiscent of the problem of African slaves in the drawing up of the American constitution. Although the slave-owning South saw slaves as property rather than humans, for purposes of representation in Congress, it was desirable to count them as real people since representation in the House is based on population (of humans). Could they have it both ways? In the tradition of compromise, it was agreed that a slave would be counted as three-fifths of a person, thereby giving the South greater representation while at the same time accepting the legal reality that a slave was not a full citizen. In the insurance world, a psychiatric patient has been only about half the worthiness of a "real" patient, showing that traditionally even a slave was worth more than a psychiatric patient.[14]

It's not that there hasn't been advocacy over the years. The Mental Health Association was founded in 1908, and National Alliance on Mental Illness has been with us for many decades. These organizations were mainly oriented toward getting better services within the public mental health systems, both inpatient and outpatient, for the more chronic and persistent mentally ill who have been with us well before there was even health insurance for medical/surgical populations.

But even with advocacy from these organizations, support has steadily dwindled. Publicly funded psychiatric beds have been reduced, presumably because of the availability of outpatient resources and more effective psychiatric medications. Nevertheless, there is no reason to believe that medications have become more effective between 2005 and 2010 when the country saw a decline in beds from 50,509 in 2005 to 43,318 in 2010 (Modern Healthcare 2013). In 1955, there were 560,000 psychiatric beds with a population perhaps three-fifths of the United States today.

In the mid-1970s, things began to change. While the introduction of antipsychotic and antidepressant drugs came in mid-1950, there was little immediate effect on stigma. In 1970, the diagnosis of manic-depressive psychosis made its reappearance in the United States after a long absence. The reason was the introduction of lithium here (finally, after being adopted earlier by most other countries in the free world), which had the effect of legitimizing the diagnosis as a medical problem rather than a nasty name we called people. As explained in chapter 10, since lithium was considered "specific" (more or less) for manic depression (the bipolar name had not yet been adopted), it therefore followed that there must be some function at the level of the brain that lithium influenced.

Once again, as with Thorazine, the functions of brain and mind

---

[14] In all fairness to the insurers, it must be said that this situation was not entirely their fault. Psychiatry, as a profession, bears some of the responsibility by avoiding development of standards of treatment for the various disorders until perhaps the last twenty years, although insurance companies largely ignore them. In the days when inpatient treatment could go on for years and psychotherapy could be considered perpetual (e.g., four times weekly for each of four different family members), there's little wonder that insurance actuaries envisioned financial Armageddon.

intersected, and patients who saw this (and weren't in denial about their condition) could say to themselves, "I have a brain disorder," which they saw as somehow destigmatizing (medical problems are more acceptable than moral ones) and allowed them to go public with their disorder. Even though we no longer thought of the mentally ill as immoral, most attempts at psychotherapy during this time ended in the belief that someone was to blame for something. If it wasn't the patient, then perhaps it was the mother, father, grandmother, society, or spouse. Somebody was to blame. In the end, if it was not a brain disorder, it became a moral problem on someone's part once again (e.g., Dr. Bettelheim's "extreme situations" created largely by parents of autistics and other mentally ill persons).

While lithium, like Thorazine, was a significant advance, "cure" was a word, as in most medical conditions, that was not appropriate. Like so many treatments, lithium was miraculous for some, good to very good for many, and disappointing for others. For many patients (and their families) manic depression was a long and difficult road with many ups and downs, requiring years of effort and struggle. But it was somehow different than it had been before. It was a disease like other diseases, and with that understanding there was hope that someday, somewhere, someone might ultimately find a cure or at least some more effective treatment. Like the diabetics and the asthmatics and cancer patients, it now became legitimate to advocate for oneself and for one's illness.

In the mid-1970s, Dr. Jan Fawcett was chair of psychiatry at what is now called Rush University Medical Center in Chicago (formerly Rush Presbyterian–St. Luke's Medical Center). Several patients treated there in the early 1970s were encouraged by him to take a more active role for themselves and other patients suffering from manic-depressive illness. Although still ill, three women took the initiative and started what was then called the Manic-Depressive Association. In the mid-1970s, the very name of the organization was a bit shocking. This organization was different. It was organized and funded by patients who actually suffered from the illness. I somehow stumbled upon a pamphlet somewhere announcing a meeting that was being held in the basement meeting room of the What's Cooking restaurant in Lincolnwood, a suburb near the northwestern city limit of Chicago. Up to that point in my career, I had never heard of any person or group of persons openly refer to themselves as manic depressives, which really was, at the time, a term of insult. The very thought of such a thing seemed to me improbable. I had no idea what to expect. My recollection is that the year was 1979.

In those days, except for alcoholics in AA meetings who used only first names, for patients to talk about their diagnoses and mental illnesses in a public forum was unheard of. Psychiatric diagnoses were extremely stigmatizing, and patients spent most of their time trying to deny whatever it was they had. Listening to them speak about themselves and their experiences publicly was an education. Hearing them talk about their medications and doctors in a positive and appreciative manner was downright shocking since this was a time in which the antipsychiatry movement was most influential. Psychiatrists were considered particularly sinful for "labeling" people with imaginary diagnoses designed to suppress free speech and incarcerate those who protested the ills of society. Psychiatrists used drugs to inflict "chemical lobotomies" on their "victims."

How bad was it? It was so bad that even psychiatrists didn't appreciate what these ladies were doing for the profession and for other psychiatric patients then and now. In fact, apart from the very significant support given these patients by Dr. Fawcett and some others at Rush, reception by the psychiatric profession at large was, I discovered at this meeting, rather chilly. The idea of patient advocacy, by the patients themselves, was not welcomed for some reason by most psychiatrists they'd encountered. It was also, they said, very unusual for a psychiatrist to actually come to a patient-run meeting at the restaurant, which was the only meeting place in those early years. Apart from Dr. Fawcett and a few others at Rush, I was apparently among the first. Only six or seven years later (1986), they became a national organization and were soon receiving the attention of major figures in academic psychiatry in addition to Jan Fawcett.

It was difficult to understand why they were having difficulty getting support from other psychiatrists early on. These were patients who'd had treatment both in hospitals and in the office. Most felt their medications had been central to their recovery and an essential part of their treatment even if they weren't fully recovered. They were positive about and supported research in psychiatry at every level, biological and psychological. They appreciated what we did and said so publicly. Psychiatrists became invited speakers at many future meetings. There was great interest in the latest research, pharmacologic and otherwise. They complained to insurance companies about the double standard in coverage. At a time when almost every public utterance about psychiatry was negative, why were we not embracing them?

The problem with psychiatrists was twofold: The 1960s and 1970s had been a period of revolutionary social change. Civil rights struggles, women's rights issues, and Vietnam War protests were all part of and helped drive the process of social change. The war in Vietnam precipitated a youth movement that questioned all traditional authority. American society became polarized for a time between what was called the "establishment" on one side and forces of the "antiestablishment" on the other. Many psychiatrists identified themselves with political causes and identified themselves as antiestablishment.

Also, much of psychiatry was seen as establishment, as in state hospitals, commitment laws, and definitions of mental illness sanctioned by the state. These were seen as manifestations of "Big Brother's" effort to control the antiestablishment types through psychiatric incarceration, "powerful" psychiatric drugs, shock treatments, and, if one were particularly defiant, lobotomy.

The film (and book) One Flew Over the Cuckoo's Nest was a good example of the mood of the time. In the film version, the Jack Nicholson character is a petty criminal who essentially fakes psychiatric symptoms because he feels life in a mental hospital would be preferable to prison. In the quintessential Jack Nicholson role, his character likes to push the envelope and stir things up and is somewhat dismayed by how well the patients put up with the "system." The patients become emblematic of the oppressed and powerless minorities that the establishment has a vested interest in subduing, and he decides he's going to lead them in revolt. Symbolic of establishment authority is Nurse Ratchet. He's drawn into a power struggle with her and she with him. It's understood in the film that there's really nothing psychiatrically wrong with the Jack Nicholson character (other than his real but charming sociopathy), and the "real" patients know it. The plot is driven by the fact that Nurse Ratchet (establishment) is offended by the challenge to her authority that he (antiestablishment) represents. She counters with the evil triad. First, the medication fails to suppress his defiant exuberance. She then counters with electroconvulsive therapy, which seems to work for a time but then fails to eradicate his independent spirit. Finally, in her pleadings with the doctors (who never interact with him but listen only to her) that she is desperately trying to help this poor soul, she refers him for lobotomy, which, of course, transforms him into a vegetable. The establishment wins, and the antiestablishment types lose in this classic tale of evil winning out over good. While psychiatrists are still complaining about the film, reviewers Gene Siskel and Roger Ebert correctly saw it as an allegory reflecting the mood of the times about authority in general, with psychiatry as a convenient vehicle.

Most of the more vocal groups that psychiatrists were hearing about in the years before 1979 supported antipsychiatry sentiments, and what organizing was being done at the time was by patients angry about being "labeled" (i.e., given a psychiatric diagnosis) or treated, presumably against their will. I was especially active in the Illinois Psychiatric Society at the time, and, when I asked other psychiatrists about the Manic-Depressive Association, most had either never heard about them or thought they were another organization of disgruntled patients not much different from organizations like Citizens Against Psychiatric Assault, organized by psychiatry's arch adversary, the Church of Scientology (L. Ron Hubbard, Tom Cruise, and so on) who were busy calling psychiatrists before their "tribunal" to confess their crimes against humanity. I'd be surprised if anyone ever showed up at these "tribunals," but stranger things have happened.

Illinois's Mental Health Code, revised in 1979, started with the assumption that most psychiatrists, hospitals, and parents were up to no good (or at best were acting paternalistically, thereby trampling on human rights). The new code demanded strict adherence to a model that supported the notion that everyone really was out to immorally rob patients of their constitutional rights. Confidentiality laws, when originally conceived, were attempting to protect patients from having their information and diagnoses used against them by employers, ex-spouses, ex-lovers, and the news media, among others. The unintended consequence, however, was that the families and parents of very ill patients (the only ones who might truly care about these patients' welfare) could go for months or years without knowledge of a patient's whereabouts or condition, or if they were alive or dead.

If a patient with a head injury comes to a hospital confused or comatose, no one questions that calling family members for information and feedback about that patient's condition is humane and medically necessary. If a psychiatric patient is brought to a hospital by police or by ambulance in a confused and psychotic state, unless the patient signs something specifically giving consent, the hospital is not allowed to acknowledge that the person is even there as a patient, much less get history or give information to the family. This is the case even if it was the family who called the ambulance! Because the patient is psychotic and frightened, not only does he refuse to sign a consent to speak to family, but the patient is unlikely to sign anything at all for any reason. Speaking to a family member criminalizes the doctor or hospital (a felonious offense) even though history in this case is medically necessary. We can order an MRI for $2,500 but can't make a 50-cent phone call to his mother. The allies of Dr. Szasz were in control. Mental illness was indeed mythical. Patients could be "liberated" from the family's malevolent control or their "schizophrenogenic mothers." While one can acknowledge that there are probably a few mothers capable of generating unwanted angst in their children, schizophrenia is another matter.

The other problem limiting psychiatry's acceptance of this kind of advocacy by patients had to do with the lingering influence of psychoanalysis and the schism between the biological and psychological orientations in the profession. While psychiatrists like Eric Kandel, mentioned in chapter 10, were hoping to find common ground and an integrated scientific language, rapprochement was still a distant dream.

Psychoanalytically oriented practitioners whom I spoke to were threatened by a group of patients who unashamedly accepted a medical model of treatment and etiology, which they saw as in error (patients were in denial or reacting to guilt) and which posed down the line (managed care at this time a mere gleam in the insurance carrier's eye) a potential threat to their understanding of the human mind and how to treat its illness. The Manic-Depressive Association, encouraged by Dr. Fawcett, saw most major mental illnesses as brain dysfunction. The differences were apparently irreconcilable.

My own "up close and personal" encounter with the antipsychiatry crowd occurred on Monday, July 6, 1986, when I appeared on a local talk show. In May 1986, I began a term as president of the Illinois Psychiatric Society. On Friday, July 3, Dr. Pat Staunton notified me that I should go on the show and represent Illinois psychiatry since I was now president.

Besides, no one else was available (or foolish enough) to do it. As is typical of shows like this, the issue wasn't education of any kind or a discussion of current issues of public interest. The issue was shock entertainment. The guests that day were two "victims" of psychiatric assault, one of whom had written a book about how he'd been hospitalized against his will and given drugs! The other was a woman who'd been hospitalized as a child for about ten years because she claimed she'd had a few "out of body" experiences, which, as everyone knew, were "perfectly normal."

Her father was a psychiatric social worker but somehow thought she was sick enough to tolerate her being in a hospital somewhere for almost a decade. These two apparently made the rounds of talk shows around the country and had their presentation honed. I learned later on a PBS discussion about the ethics of "ambush interviews" that I'd been, well … ambushed. In an ambush one party has a specific agenda and a specific presentation with specific allegations and/or complaints about something or someone. Arraigned against these complainants is some poor fool who is notified a few hours before about the request for an appearance but is given no information about what the issues are and no time for preparation even if the issues to be "discussed" were known. I didn't get to see any records. I couldn't even read the man's book. The goal, I had to realize, was shock entertainment and not serious discussion of anything. This was not Ted Koppel or Charlie Rose. I tried to say as little as possible and let the others ramble on. The theme was that no one should ever be treated against their will. Psychiatrists just liked to lock people up so they could send bills and wield control over people.

An unusual event happened just before intermission. As the program was running, someone in New York on the Staten Island ferry had a long knife or a sword of some kind and was attacking some of the passengers. As it was reported in the news flash, this person had been seen at a New York psychiatric clinic, either that day or recently, and not forcibly hospitalized. Now the victims, prepared for these situations, began to complain that psychiatrists were at fault for not hospitalizing this particular patient. Then came the phoned-in comments and questions. The first caller had been hospitalized against her will sometime in the recent past. However, she went on to say that it was the right thing to do in her case because, when she got better, she realized she was indeed out of her mind, and someone needed to help her even if she, at that moment, disagreed. As this woman was talking, the host gave a disgruntled look to one of the engineers that clearly conveyed her displeasure at someone making a positive comment on the air, and the woman was cut off. She was looking for complaints, not praise. The whole experience was embarrassing, but I survived.

The medical treatment of psychiatric disorders is itself stigmatizing. In 1972, George McGovern ran against Richard Nixon for president and chose Missouri senator Thomas Eagleton as his vice presidential candidate. Shortly after the announcement, it was discovered that Senator Eagleton had been treated for depression some years prior and had been treated with electroconvulsive therapy (ECT). ECT was seen as a lobotomy equivalent in those days. Even though he had recovered and was a fairly accomplished senator, the fact that he had undergone treatment with ECT torpedoed his candidacy. Senator McGovern felt forced to remove him and pick a new candidate. It was his only choice since from that point forward there was constant questioning about having a "crazy person" just a heartbeat away from the presidency. Every other aspect of Eagleton's life was of no consequence. The only important fact was that he received ECT, and that was unacceptable. Had he been from New York and treated with psychoanalysis, it would have been a nonissue since "everyone" (who was anyone) in New York was in analysis (only a slight exaggeration). There was nothing in the history of Senator Eagleton to suggest he was any crazier (i.e., irrational or lacking in judgment) than New Yorkers in psychoanalysis and was probably much less so.

Eagleton's problem was that he was from Missouri, and he was simply interested in getting better. He was treated very successfully by Washington University (St. Louis) doctors who were generally not inclined to long periods of psychotherapy, as the favored form of treatment for a major depression. After being pushed off the ticket, he remained in the US Senate for several terms, and his mental health was never an issue. In ways it turned out to be a blessing since Nixon won in a landslide anyway.

Before I leave the topic of stigma, I'd like to reference a 1991 film portrayal of acute mania (bipolar mania), which was the best I'd ever seen, including the more recent film Silver Linings Playbook, which was also quite a good (and sympathetic) portrayal of bipolar mania. The Madness of King George is about King George III, who was the British king who presided over the loss of the American colonies in the American Revolutionary War. While I can't speak with authority about just what symptoms the king really displayed historically, I can say that the portrayal of mania (the king's madness) in the film was accurate and masterful. In the end, however, we're led to believe that the madness wasn't really "madness" at all, but a behavioral manifestation of a metabolic disorder known as porphyria. Since it wouldn't be right to suggest that insanity runs in the English royal family, porphyria, which presumably made this king mad, is okay. If porphyria is an inherited disorder and can make one develop a clinical picture that looks exactly like a bipolar manic, why is the porphyria less stigmatizing than bipolar mania? I personally doubt that the king actually had porphyria. If the film portrayal was accurate, he was bipolar manic.

Electroconvulsive Therapy

When I mention ECT to a patient or a family, I've learned from considerable experience to expect almost anything from shocked disbelief and anger to thankful praise. Despite seventy-five years of relatively safe and highly effective results (comparing favorably to many other medical procedures), ECT somehow remains controversial. Some of the controversy is a lingering political issue left over from the 1960s, 1970s, and early 1980s. At the time, "medical" treatment in psychiatry was regarded as a synonym for assault and battery, whether one used ECT or prescribed medication.

In the heyday of psychotherapy for major psychiatric conditions, treating someone with ECT was considered by many psychiatrists as, at best, superficial, if not downright barbaric, because we weren't getting at the "root cause" of the illness. One of the unfortunate effects of reinterpreted psychoanalytic thinking in psychiatry was the belief that we could know the root causes of major psychiatric disorders when we really could not (there's a difference between a root cause and a precipitating event). Because we didn't know the "cause" of many cancers, diabetes, or lupus (though that's changing rapidly as we speak), that didn't mean physicians couldn't treat those conditions fairly effectively. Conversely, even if we postulate and/or prove a genetic cause and identify the specific gene (or collection of genes), that doesn't mean we can do anything about it, though it is a great beginning and is exactly what's happening in psychiatric research today.

As residents at the University of Illinois Neuropsychiatric Institute in 1966 to 1967, we used ECT only one time, and that was at my request. Outcome and safety data, even then, supported its use in what today would be considered a bipolar depressed or major depressive patient who had been in the hospital for over six months and treated with medication and daily psychotherapy sessions. Several attempts to discharge him resulted in rapid decompensation and recurrence of suicidal preoccupation. My supervisors for this patient, most of whom were analysts or in analytic training, allowed me to go ahead with the procedure but couldn't instruct me in its use, because they'd never done it.

There was one faculty psychiatrist who was trained at Washington University in St. Louis (also in Chicago for analytic training) whose task it was to teach the residents about psychotropic drugs. He was familiar with ECT, so we were able to make an attempt, though it was very awkward. We did have an ancient ECT machine somewhere, but at first no one was able to locate it. On the day of the first treatment, the procedure got delayed by at least an hour, because the anesthesiologist didn't know how to get to the Neuropsychiatric Institute, having become lost in the tunnels connecting our building with other University of Illinois hospital buildings. To say that we in psychiatry were disconnected from the medical mainstream was an obvious understatement.

It's not that the faculty at the University of Illinois were against doing ECT for the right patient; it was just that it had been a decade or more since they'd been able to find that right patient. Schizophrenia could somehow be understood in the framework of a psychoanalytic developmental psychology, but manic depression (bipolar disorders), with all those ups and downs of mood and periods of wellness, did not lend itself to psychodynamic interpretation despite Freud's blessing in Mourning and Melancholia. The result was that, in the psychoanalytic world of the 1950s and 1960s, manic-depressive disorders were diagnoses that European doctors used, but the more enlightened thinkers in the United States did not.

Fortunately, my ECT patient, a graduate student at the University of Chicago, did well with ECT and was out of the hospital within about three weeks. Having been out of school for seven months, he could not immediately return to the university but was well enough to go home. He was overjoyed to be out of the hospital and feeling better. He seemed to care less about the political implications.

Political implications? What political implications?

Only psychiatric treatments had political implications in 1967; the juxtaposition of race and ECT required further "analysis." The patient was an African American[15] from rural Mississippi, and from social psychiatry lectures and readings we understood that in the United States in the 1960s, the upper and upper-middle classes seeking psychiatric treatment were likely to get psychotherapy, and lower-class whites and African Americans were more likely to get "somatic treatments" (i.e., drugs and ECT). And what did this mean? The implication was that the poorer classes were either being mistreated or receiving inferior treatment. After all, we believed that those with financial resources (or insurance) had more choices than those without so presumably would more often choose or be referred for psychotherapy. It was in too many cases an either/or world based on incompatible belief systems.

In an analytic program we learned to explore not only the presumed transference (unconscious distortions in the patient controlled or induced by early trauma) phenomena in patients, but also the presumed countertransference (i.e., the unconscious distortions and prejudices, possibly racial, in the psychiatrist, which was why a personal analysis for the doctor was always recommended) in order to treat the situation as objectively as possible. This patient was treated with daily psychotherapy

---

[15] Father was born in 1914, so in 1966 he was fifty-two years old. Since he was born at home of illiterate immigrant parents, he never got an official birth certificate. The only document my grandparents had was a baptismal certificate on which was contained his date of baptism but not his birthdate. When it came time to enroll him in school, a birth certificate was required. Barely speaking English, his parents somehow didn't find a way to get the required document, so he didn't go to school until he was picked up by police at age nine on the street as a truant. Nevertheless, he managed to graduate from Crane Technical High School (one of two or three "tech" schools in Chicago at the time) in 1931 at age seventeen. Like many children of immigrants, then and now, he found mathematics to be an area not requiring major proficiency in English. After graduation he worked where he could during the daytime and began a night program in electrical engineering at the Illinois Institute of Technology with a projected graduation date of 1939. He never made it that far, but, with the approach of World War II, work as a draftsman became plentiful.

(Monday through Friday) for six months, but the patient didn't seem to appreciate the insights he was gaining and just wanted to get better and go home. This patient was no Woody Allen. Few are.

We prescribed medication. By 1966, medication for our inpatients was not unusual, and cost (time in the hospital) was never an issue. After all, the patients were ill enough to be hospitalized. Did we unconsciously select this patient for ECT because he was poor and black? That was a tough one. Yes, he was from a poor economic background, but he was, after all, on a full scholarship at the University of Chicago, and even in 1966 one still had to be fairly accomplished to get into University of Chicago, much less have them give you money to be there. So his prospects for the middle class seemed pretty good, although he had a rather down-home manner. Since racism can be a powerful unconscious phenomenon, one can never absolutely rule it out as a factor. On the other hand, I don't believe my supervisor and I underestimated the effect of the culture shock he experienced by suddenly finding himself in a very alien environment (Hyde Park, Chicago) far away from his rural Mississippi home, though he already was a college graduate. It was very likely a significant precipitating factor and worked on in psychotherapy for over six months. But sending him home in his present condition, even after six months, was not an option we could safely exercise.

ECT did not fit a psychoanalytic paradigm, and any beneficial effect could not be explained. Like many Hollywood films, some analysts saw ECT as battery of guilt-laden depressed patients, which worked by giving them the punishment they already thought they deserved. Depression was interpreted as anger turned against the self. One couldn't absolutely say it wasn't racism, but I perhaps naively believed I was simply doing what physicians have always done, alleviating patient suffering and getting him better. The African American residents in my residency class (two of the six in my year) seemed to support my suggestion and were impressed by the outcome in his case.

Prior to the time this African American patient was admitted (and paralleling his treatment), my own father developed, for the first time in his life that anyone knew of, very severe depression. His rather dramatic symptoms began somewhere between the time of my graduation from medical school and the start of residency training a year later (one did internships in those days). The condition probably started at least a year before med school graduation but presented more with vague physical symptoms. It became more severe while I was interning in Los Angeles. Shortly after my return to Chicago, he became too ill to work.

It was a rather humbling experience, because everything was done to get him seen by the "best" program in the area, where he was recommended for inpatient treatment. Upon admission, the estimated length of stay for his condition was given as two years. Suicide did not appear to be an issue at any time during his illness, the most severe portion of which lasted about eighteen months, during which time he was completely unable to work or do anything else.

As a patient, Father was uncooperative, even hostile to the treatment process, and spent most of his treatment time telling his doctor that there was nothing wrong with him. He wanted to leave the hospital to return to work, which at that time was, of course, not possible. Since this was a psychotherapy-oriented program, the relationship here was strictly between the doctor and the patient (it was presumed that talking to the family would not be well received by the patient, who would then not speak spontaneously to the psychiatrist) and not between the doctor and the patient's wife or family. This reality did not endear the doctor to Mother, who was not a patient woman and expected at least weekly reports.

As it happened, a longtime neighborhood friend of mine, Dr. James Jordan, was interning at the hospital where Father was being treated and would visit him from time to time. Since they had known each other for at least the past ten years, Father felt comfortable telling him what he told his family: that the doctor was crazier than he was and this "so-called treatment" would not work. There was nothing "mental" about his problem. He simply needed to return to work. Jim said he was struck by the dramatic weight loss, agitation, and visible transformation in general appearance from the person he had seen and known before. He was impressed by how "sick" Father appeared despite his protestations.

After four to six weeks of this, both Father and Mother got fed up, and she urged him (more like ordered him) to sign out of the hospital, which didn't take much convincing on his part, although taking any action was agonizing for him. She felt he was "sick" and was making no progress, and the doctor there wasn't acting like any doctor she'd ever dealt with. Since she worked at a hospital (as a switchboard operator and receptionist at Loretto Hospital, which had a psychiatric unit), she felt she knew a doctor when she saw (or spoke to) one. For his part, Father felt like so many psychiatric patients, that there was nothing wrong with him. He took his inability to earn a living now as a moral failing, which made him, if possible, even more depressed.

There were at least three other serious attempts at treatment, in addition to various antidepressants, all of which failed. It followed a pattern: After his first hospitalization of about a month, he came home and was better for a few days. Then his agitation would build again and eventually got to a point that Mother felt she couldn't take it anymore, and he'd get hospitalized again. Same routine. Same complaints. Same outcome.

However, his depression was so severe and cognitive capacities so impaired that at the last hospital the psychiatrist actually gave him a diagnosis of "organic brain disorder," which in effect was a diagnosis of presenile dementia, since he was only fifty-three years old and had no history of brain trauma. Discharge instructions were to apply for Social Security disability, and nothing else could be done for this poor demented man.

In old-fashioned descriptive (medical) psychiatry is found a term used to describe depressions so severe that they resemble dementias but resolve if the depression remits or is successfully treated—a "curable dementia," if you will. It was called "pseudo-dementia."

Since Father never had or never admitted to suicidal thoughts, the next program we brought him to (after months of interminable misery at home) recommended something new: a day hospital program. He was completely nonfunctional and had lost forty pounds. As in many serious depressions, he could not sleep at night, felt agitated and horrible in the morning, and couldn't leave the house. If he could leave the house in the morning, he argued, he would have gone to work. Of course, since he couldn't, he never attended the day hospital program. Now he was "uncooperative, noncompliant, and didn't want to get better!" Hopelessness and misery were the order of the day, and he was intolerable to be around since he made everyone around him feel as miserable as he did. I was busy and found reasons not to visit. Such is the fate of those who attempt to live with or visit someone this depressed. By this time I had just given ECT to my patient and was impressed with the result. No one he'd seen the entire year of active treatment so far had recommended it.

He failed all the "best" programs, so Mother went out and found a neighborhood psychiatrist who hospitalized him locally and gave him ECT, and after more than sixteen months out of work (and receiving disability checks), he was back working maybe four weeks later (after about a week of post-ECT hypomania, during which time this extremely frugal man thought a Cadillac was in his future) and worked for another eighteen years before he retired.

His was the classical melancholia, exactly as described by Hippocrates, circa 425 BC, which, in 1966 to 1967, had more or less completely disappeared from the psychiatric radar screen at the "best" training programs. In 1973, I wrote an account of this experience, which was published in the American Journal of Psychiatry (D'Agostino 1975). The title of the article was "Depression: Schism in Contemporary Psychiatry." Their willingness to accept this single case report for publication in one of psychiatry's more prestigious journals suggests that the editor also thought it was interesting enough that the "best" training programs in the country had stopped teaching the use of one of the most effective treatments in medicine.

For both my African American patient and my father, one really couldn't say whether in perhaps another three, five, seven, or ten more years of therapy they would not have gotten better. Could psychotherapy do it? How long does one wait? Spontaneous remissions do occur for who knows what reasons. Let's say another five or six years of 24-7 in hell. Would waiting that long be worth it? What one can say for sure is that they would have been considerably poorer and return to full-time work or school very slowly, if ever. It was more than fortunate that he worked for a major manufacturing company that made printing presses (Father made blueprints) and had great 1960s health insurance. Today, under managed care, since he said he wasn't suicidal and was "noncompliant with treatment," he may not have gotten any treatment at all and saved the insurance company a lot of money but cost the taxpayers many years of Social Security payments, not to mention potential Medicare expenses. In my experience, once someone is on SSI, it takes enormous drive and confidence in a patient to give that up for the uncertainty of competitive employment, which is why getting patients better as fast as possible has both prognostic and economic implications.

Another source of trouble with psychiatry's use of ECT is that, until recently, to the general public it seemed like overkill. Concerns about potential side effects like memory loss (which will occur temporarily in most patients to some degree), dramatic personality changes (never seen by me in forty-five years), or "brain damage" (an unchallenged claim for many years) seem like excessive risk for a problem that may seem trivial or merely "psychological" (a synonym for imaginary or not real) to relatives and friends. In the case of my father, was he "sick," or was it "psychological"?

Some have images in their head about barbaric torture derived from the name often used for the procedure "shock therapy," which does not conjure up pleasant images. The use of unmodified ECT in the early years (ECT without benefit of anesthesia and muscle relaxants) was indeed "shocking" to observers and potentially dangerous to patients. Imagine observing any major surgery today without general anesthesia, going back to those old favorites, alcohol and opium. I can guarantee the reader would find it "shocking."

The procedure involves the induction of a grand mal seizure, which critics have argued is an abnormal event for the brain. Of course, most major surgical procedures are not exactly "natural" events for the body, as the multitudes of deaths via postsurgical infections and other complications for the past six thousand years (of recorded history) bear witness. Surgeries have complications with unavoidable frequency even in the best hands, and nonpsychiatric medications have side effects, as well, sometimes serious side effects like death (call 1-800-BAD DRUG and see).

All patients, surgical or ECT, sign consents based on a probability gamble, which goes something like this: What's the danger or negative outcome to me if I don't have the procedure versus if I have it? There are potential negatives on both sides of the decision, but if the risk of refusing the treatment is lower than the risk of doing it, the patient (and the doctor) should reconsider going forward unless a very compelling reason for doing it anyway can be made. The reason ECT looks like it has higher risk than most surgical procedures (which it does not) is that some regard surgical disorders as more "serious" than psychiatric ones. By this comparison, the risk–benefit analysis looks better for surgery. In the case of a bowel obstruction, a dissecting aneurysm, or a tubal pregnancy, of course it is. In many cosmetic and other elective procedures, however, it's not. This is not a way of saying that cosmetic or elective surgical procedures shouldn't be done or that they're particularly dangerous, only that the risk–benefit analysis favors ECT in many scenarios. Severe depression, an active bipolar condition, or psychosis is quite serious, can constitute a medical emergency of the first rank, and can be associated with serious negative outcomes if untreated or if unsuccessfully treated.

ECT doesn't work in everyone all the time, but I can't think of too many medical or surgical procedures that do (e.g., surgery for back pain, many procedures for the treatment of cancer and heart disease, among others). Like every other procedure in medicine, ECT has indications. There are plenty of psychiatric disorders for which ECT is not indicated. In the 1960s and 1970s, there were active attempts to ban ECT in various states, especially California. The issue here involved the legitimacy of any biological treatment, drug or otherwise, for any psychiatric condition, since psychiatric disorders had nothing to do with the brain.

It was called the antipsychiatry movement, and it had three primary beliefs (Kandel,1998). The first was that mental illness was not an objective behavioral or biochemical phenomenon but a "label" whose function was social control of those who challenged prevailing norms. The second was that madness had a truth of its own that needs to be expressed. Lastly, under the right circumstances, psychosis could be a healing process and should not be pharmacologically "suppressed" (Porter 1997). This view's chief spokesperson in the United States was Thomas Szasz, a psychoanalyst whose book, The Myth of Mental Illness, was mentioned in chapter 10. The antipsychiatry groups were particularly active in California and were successful in limiting the use of ECT.

The state of California didn't ban ECT outright but set up so many impediments to treatment as to effectively eliminate much of it in the state. The city of Berkeley outright banned it, seeing it as patient abuse in every case. Historically, for a city council to ban a medical procedure based not on medical evidence but on strictly political grounds is very unusual. When I was a fellow at UCLA in the late 1960s and in the US Navy stationed in California in 1969 to 1971, it became apparent to me that patients who could afford to travel and had decent insurance coverage simply sought treatment in Nevada and Arizona until the political winds shifted again. Meanwhile, at that time in history, trying to argue that medical insurance should cover "mythical" conditions was quite challenging. Nevertheless, in my career, I've never seen insurance, managed or not, question the legitimacy of ECT, since it gets people better quicker and is cost-effective from an insurance point of view.

The acceptance of ECT by the general public in 2018 is far greater than in the 1960s and 1970s. Patients today are used to public debate over a variety of medical/surgical procedures and are less likely to see ECT as battery, even if they elect not to have it. However, the 1960s Berkeley mentality persists and frequently pops up in the cinema. The 2010 film *Changeling* is a recent example. As with many films these days, it is alleged to be "based on true events." Years ago virtually all films were listed in the credits as fictitious and "any resemblance to persons living or dead is purely coincidental." Now most new films seem to be "based on true events." The devil here is in the words "true (kinda sorta) events."

In *Changeling*, Angelina Jolie plays the mother of a nine- or ten-year-old child who disappears one day. She goes to the police for help in recovering him. After some time, they call her to say that they've found her son so come and get him. The boy they offer as her son is not her son but meets the general description of a ten-year-old white kid, so the Los Angeles Police allegedly close the case. When she persists in saying the boy they've given her is not her son, they somehow conclude that she's delusional and have her committed to a psychiatric hospital (which is somehow in collusion with the bad guys). Here she's given ECT, basically as a kind of punishment for persisting in her "delusion," which here is her refusal to recognize her own son. The child is portrayed as an abused runaway from the Midwest who finds himself in need of care and feeding so is, however improbably, willing to say that the Angelina Jolie character is his mother.

The problem (among others) is that this all happens in 1927 Los Angeles, and ECT is still eleven years away from being invented. Since the film is "based on true events," the film would like us to believe that something like this (a child kidnapping ring, allied with corrupt police, connected to a psychiatric hospital that locked up the mothers of kidnapped and murdered children) happened in 1920s Los Angeles. Maybe it did, but one can be quite certain that ECT could not have been part of that story. This raises the question of why it was included in the film. One wonders what the filmmaker is trying to tell us. Did they feel the script needed a few more lurid details they felt the story lacked? Are the kidnapping and murdering of children not lurid enough? In this context once again, psychiatrists treat people who are not mentally ill (conditions that do not exist, in fact) for criminal purposes, with Hollywood's most visible and dramatically portrayed symbols of mental abuse: psychiatric hospitals and electroconvulsive therapy.

It would be inappropriate to exit a discussion about ECT without a few remarks about the brain damage allegations. I will get to the issue, but I hope you will allow me a brief digression.

Obvious brain damage occurs in a variety of activities about which for years there has been little or no debate. In the sport of boxing the goal is to "knock out" one's opponent. Knocking out someone is not easy to do and can be accomplished only by inflicting damage to someone's brain, usually by contusing it against the rigid structure of the skull. Think of the brain as a kind of soft Bavarian Jell-O mold, which, when suddenly bashed or jostled, crashes against the skull, causing damage enough for the person to lose consciousness secondary to trauma, swelling, and bleeding in the brain.

Getting repeated blows to the head, as occurs in thousands of football games each week in the fall, is cause for many concussions, some deaths, and major legal actions currently under way between the National Football League (NFL) and former players showing signs of dementia in their fifties. According to a course I took on traumatic brain injuries at the annual APA convention in 2013, the incidence of formally diagnosed dementia in NFL players under the age of fifty is one in fifty. In the general population of men under age fifty, that diagnosis occurs in only one per thousand, a twenty-fold increase. Beyond age fifty, it's even higher, and about 30 percent of all NFL players can expect some demonstrable brain damage. Even in soccer, "headers" involve being hit in the head by a soccer ball traveling at great speed as an intentional display of playing skill, although most concussions in soccer occur from players crashing into one another.

While the American Medical Association years ago called for a ban on the sport of boxing, the state of California has yet to act. One would have to suppose that the entertainment value and income potential far outweigh the risks since there remain more than enough candidates in all three sports. Football is more popular than ever. While I believe boxing should be banned as a sport in the United States, I do not feel the same about soccer or football. There are risks in many activities, and, once the risks are known, people have to make up their own minds. But one can easily see that putting a brain at risk for entertainment trumps putting it at risk for therapeutics.

Nevertheless, the reasonable person and even many physicians find it difficult to believe than running an electrical current through the brain and causing a seizure is not harmful to brain tissue. Isn't that what we do when we kill someone in an electric chair? Is this an issue of dose—50,000 volts versus a few joules? Is it the seizure per se that threatens the brain, or are there other factors?

For many years, even among psychiatrists, there was an assumption of some damage, but the severity of the conditions treated were such that it seemed worth the risk since the only evidence of damage was anterograde (from the first treatment forward) and some retrograde (the period before treatment started) memory loss, which was almost always very temporary. As noted in the case of my father, his brain appeared to work much better after ECT than before. In fact, it cured (a word seldom used in psychiatry or medicine) his "dementia," as well as his depression. It's important to be clear here. Before ECT his brain wasn't working well, since on examination he seemed demented. Except for mild memory loss, which was very temporary, his brain worked better after he had ECT. Depression had a negative effect on his brain. However, it is also important to note that completely ruling out the possibility of some damage (if that's the cause of the memory loss), however mild, in a minority of cases is simply not possible. But being seriously depressed and untreated is not exactly brain enriching either, and the assumption that schizophrenia, bipolar disorders, and serious major depressions have innocuous effects in the brain is no longer tenable (Gildengers et al. 2013; Bourne et al. 2013; Nunes et al. 2007; Diniz et al. 2013; Wong et al. 2008).

Complications are possible in a multitude of medical procedures done on a daily basis across the country. Doctors minimize risk by following safety procedures, which render ECT and other procedures as safe as they can be, but no one that I know of is giving 100 percent guarantees in any specialty. There are complications occurring daily in cosmetic surgeries, some of them quite serious, but no city council that I know of in California has banned cosmetic surgery. A case in point was that of comedian Totie Fields, who went into a Miami hospital in 1976 for an "eye and chin lift" (Miami news 1976). She came out of the hospital missing one of her legs and eventually died. She developed a blood clot with even a "minor" procedure. Something similar happened to comedian Joan Rivers with a "minor office procedure."

About ten years ago, a family friend, believing her arms were too fat, decided to have the fat removed through a cosmetic procedure. This was a procedure she'd saved for for several years. I have to presume that she signed an informed consent document and was willing to assume whatever risk was involved since she regarded her fat arms as an abhorrent physical characteristic. Something went wrong during surgery, and today, ten years later, she remains in a coma (her brain is irrevocably damaged) and requires total care in a nursing home. These things happen with some frequency, and she did give consent for the procedure. In this case, what was the risk of not having surgery? Answer: the emotional pain of having fat arms. As of this writing, California has not seen fit to ban liposuction.

The main threat to the brain, whether by heart attack or stroke or seizure, is lack of oxygen. Unless the tissue itself is damaged by concussion or contusion (e.g., a bullet or spear or blow to the head by a 240-pound linebacker running at full speed), a seizure is not, of itself, damaging. Bleeding into the brain or frankly damaged neurons is damaging to the brain. A grand mal seizure is many neurons depolarizing at once so the oxygen requirements for the duration of the seizure are high, which is why patients are hyperoxygenated and oxygen saturation is monitored before, during, and after a seizure. As noted in chapter 6, muscle relaxants have virtually eliminated fractures as a cause of concern.

Electricity levels in ECT are very small and administered staccato-like called brief pulse wave (similar to an antilock braking system) to precipitate a seizure using about one-seventh of the energy of a continuous or sinewave stimulus (Abrams 1997; Abrams and Essman 1982). As few as two to four joules of energy have been successful in achieving clinical improvement for seizures (Small, Small, and Milstein 1986). Muscle-relaxing agents eliminate 90 percent or more of the motor activity, and the whole procedure is over in about three to five minutes. So, with all these newfangled modifications, how damaging is it? These issues have been debated for decades in literally thousands of publications and are still not completely settled. However, there are studies supporting the notion of some good things for the brain. The most recent studies using sophisticated neuroimaging techniques show neurogenesis (i.e., growth of new cells, especially in the hippocampal region), which seem to reverse the neuronal loss seen in conditions like depression (Wong). Recent animal studies have also shown increases in dendrite growth (connectivity between cells) in the frontal and prefrontal areas of the brain after repeated ECTs (Wong). Eric Kandel (2005) believed that if we took the time to look, we'd likely find negative changes in the brain in psychiatric illness, and now we do. The notion that many mental illnesses might actually be harmful to one's brain comes as a shock, even (surprisingly) to many psychiatrists who for many years apparently thought they were actually working on the patient's soul.

"Powerful" Psychotropic Drugs

Psychotropic drugs are also part of the trouble with psychiatry. There has been, over the years, considerable reluctance to acknowledge that psychotropic drugs have any useful role to play in the treatment of psychiatric disorders regardless of what clinical practice and the evidence has shown. "Chemical lobotomy" was how some disparagingly referred to it. Especially ominous is the use of the word "powerful" when juxtaposed with (psychotropic) drugs, which I'm sure I've heard hundreds of times on radio and TV over my forty-five-plus years in the profession. The same is not true for most other drugs. For example, when a pain relief product is being advertised, one usually hears the phrases "extra strength" or "powerful medicine" used as if these were qualities in a drug that consumers thought were desirable. In psychiatry, "powerful" is a pejorative term. Of course, when it comes to side effects for over-the-counter pain relievers, the "powerful medicine" is at the same time "gentle on the stomach" (i.e., the side effects are minor), lest the word "powerful" scare off potential customers. In picking a drug for treatment of a cancer or bubonic plague or AIDS, for example, does the physician prefer a "powerful" drug to kill cancer cells or plague bacteria or the human immunovirus, or the opposite, a "not very powerful" or rather weak drug? As far as public acceptance is concerned, one might suppose that the condition being treated is relevant to the argument.

Untreated, all three diseases listed above are often lethal, so using a "powerful" drug is warranted given the alternatives, and putting up with undesirable effects is worth the risk. When it comes to psychiatric disorders, which at least some believe are mythical creations of power-crazed but clever (psychiatrists take their compliments where they find them) doctors, there seems to be something particularly risky in their use. The presence of any side effect at all makes their use seem unwarranted, even though psychiatric illnesses have mortality rates in the 15 percent range (a German study I will cite below had a 25 percent mortality rate). Adding to this the fact that many of the most severely ill don't accept the reality of mental illness (in themselves), one can see more clearly why the use of psychotropic medication is so much more controversial than in most other areas in medicine.

Although all psychotropic drugs are in some way controversial, the class known as antipsychotics is at the head of the pack. Thorazine, described in chapter 8 as the first psychotropic, is an antipsychotic, The term "antipsychotic" is itself a problem because of the term "psychotic," which, right out of the box, is stigmatizing and therefore pejorative. Patients will refuse to take antipsychotics because of the name, even today. If we call them something else, like "mood stabilizers," they become more palatable. The first official mood stabilizer approved by the FDA was lithium in 1970. The primary disorders treated by mood stabilizers have, since about the late 1980s, been known as bipolar disorders. As in schizophrenia, those with bipolar disorders can become very psychotic, as well.

Besides lithium, other mood stabilizers approved for use in the United States are anticonvulsants, drugs originally approved for the treatment of epilepsy. As with aspirin (and Thorazine), drugs developed for one indication are often found useful for another. In terms of sheer numbers, however, antipsychotics represent the largest drug group approved by the FDA for use as mood stabilizers.

Antidepressants are a bit less controversial but have their problems as well. Since depression and anxiety disorders are much less stigmatizing and much more common than psychosis, public acceptance is higher. This is one of the controversies (i.e., they're presumably prescribed too much). While serving as members of the managed care committee of the American Psychiatric Association in the late 1990s, Dr. Teas and I learned that, according to Cigna health insurance claims, psychiatrists were prescribers of antidepressant drugs in only 17 percent of patients. As a psychiatrist, I do not necessarily see this as a problem, since many nonpsychiatrist physicians are competent prescribers, and many, if not most, of these patients are being seen frequently in psychotherapy, as well. The experience at Alexian

Brothers is unlikely to be so different from other medical systems where the complicated and more severe patients will usually find their way to psychiatrists.

Nevertheless, there are negatives that all psychiatrists are aware of and that should be acknowledged. As occurs in most every other specialty, there are many patients who do not respond or who do not respond well to available treatment, with or without drugs. There are still too many cases of schizophrenia or bipolar illness that are clearly chronic and persistent and many major depressive disorders that are treatment-resistant even with the best available care.

When I was a medical student in the early 1960s, there was a kind of medical student slang term, which we called the "rule of thirds." I have no reason to believe it was not used at other schools or that it's not in use today. It sprang into use for me after completing sophomore year's course in pharmacology and is applied by students generally to most drugs used in various diseases. While my memory has to do with a psychopharmacology lecture about the recently introduced Thorazine, it was much more universal. The lecturer's presentation was that we could expect an excellent response to Thorazine and other drugs in about a third of patients, a good to fair response in a third, and a fair to poor response in roughly a third. As we went through the actions and efficacy of myriad other drugs in various diseases, especially chronic diseases, it soon became apparent that the "rule of thirds" was predictive.

The Darwin–Wallace theory of evolution through natural selection is based on the premise that individuals within any species vary slightly from one another. Without variation there can be no evolution. The study of the relationship between genetics and drug response is called pharmacogenetics. The rule of thirds is a reflection of human genetic variation at the level of the receptors that drugs interact with, as well as the way a particular body metabolizes a particular drug, all controlled by genes.

In the treatment of some cancers, the study of the genetic characteristics of tumor cell types is resulting in more effective cancer-treating strategies and drugs. A better understanding of the genetics of why some mentally ill persons respond very well to psychotropic drugs and some do not will eventually be solved and better treatment developed. Obviously it is far easier to examine the genetics of a biopsied tumor cell than divine the complex genetic interactions in brain cells, which is why psychiatric and neurologic diseases are so much more difficult to study. Difficult is not the same as impossible. The Obama administration has taken the initiative to support the funding of more basic research in psychiatric/neurologic disease, because in the long run effective treatment will be less expensive than the cost of chronic care and disability.

For the moment, however, if a patient is unresponsive or under-responsive, there is often a tendency to add or change medication while both the patient and the doctor are reluctant to give something up until a new medication choice has demonstrated value. In someone who shows no benefit at all with multiple medications, and side effects from chronic medication use begin to impact a patient, there is no point in using any drug for any condition if it doesn't help. For the most treatment-resistant patients, if they cannot be maintained at home, custodial care will be necessary. However, custodial care is not easy to come by these days, and taking some patients off presumably ineffective drugs can result in the resumption of the violent and/or self-destructive behaviors that occasioned the medications in the first place.

For those who show some (less than 50 percent) benefit but lose even that when entirely off medication, the choices are difficult. When this happens, the patient and/or the family often comes to the conclusion that the medication is the cause of the problem rather than a result. Going off medication then eventually begins a new cycle of hospitalization and disability. For these patients, life can be arduous and frustrating. However, even in the patient populations who require periodic hospitalization (like the ones seen at Alexian Brothers Behavioral Health), most are reasonably functional and eventually employable, and ultimately do relatively well. Some do remarkably well, even after a major psychosis if it's not allowed to go on for too long. And those in the psychiatric population who never require hospitalization can be expected to do even better.

In 1998, author Sylvia Nasar published A Beautiful Mind, a biography of John Forbes Nash Jr., a mathematician who won the Nobel Prize in Economics in 1994. According to Nasar, "at twenty-one, the handsome, ambitious, eccentric graduate student invented what would become the most influential theory of rational human behavior in modern social science. Nash's contribution to 'Game Theory' would ultimately revolutionize the field of economics." There was a movie version starring Russell Crowe a few years later. Both the book and the film version were tastefully done, and both were sensitive portrayals of a brilliant man caught in the throes of a horrible and debilitating schizophrenic illness. The book is fifty chapters in which Nasar explores his early life in West Virginia, his college years at Princeton, and his professorship at MIT, where he becomes famous. Words like "eccentric" and "unconventional" are used to describe him premorbidly, but at around age thirty he experiences a major psychotic decomposition, which goes on for almost thirty years.

On the back book jacket of A Beautiful Mind, David Herbert Donald states, "At once a powerful and moving biography of a great mathematical genius and an important contribution to American intellectual history." It is also a powerful and moving description of schizophrenia and its effect on Nash and his family. It also gives credit to the empathy and tolerance of the mathematical community at Princeton and his friends and family for the way they stuck by him during his many years of frank psychosis, which was not an easy task.

Nash was quietly psychotic and nonviolent except when he required hospitalization, which was often. Books are always more informative than films, because the emphasis in a film is on its entertainment (i.e., financial) potential, whereas in a book the goal is more accurate historical information. Films may be forgiven for "dramatic license" or can get away with "based on true events," but historians have no such luxury. A historian may be accused of a prejudicial slant but cannot afford to become known as a writer of fiction. The film tried to portray the seriousness of his paranoid delusions and hallucinations, but the book also explored his utter inability to be a husband, as well as a parent to either of his two children, one born out of wedlock and one who also became schizophrenic. He was a sympathetic figure but someone who could do little to reciprocate the attention and care he received from his family.

In chapter 47 of A Beautiful Mind, titled "Remission," she does an excellent mini-review of the recent literature on remission in schizophrenia and discovers that remission, as Nash seems to have achieved, is not as rare as formerly thought. In a follow-up study of five hundred schizophrenic patients by a German group, about 25 percent were dead (American death rates are a bit lower), mostly by suicides. It seems that psychiatric illness—in this case, schizophrenia—has a mortality rate comparable to other relatively high-mortality diseases (Huber, Gross, and Shuttler 1980). But roughly another 25 percent were seemingly in remission and more or less functional. The suicides occurred mostly in the first ten years of illness and presumably in patients "who got well enough between acute episodes to appreciate the awfulness of what lay ahead of them and succumbed to despair." The key word here is "awfulness." Schizophrenia is not an innocuous condition.

In earlier chapters, what she reports about Nash is the fact that he responded rather well to virtually every treatment given to him during his many hospitalizations, including both antipsychotic medications and insulin coma (see chapter 6), which he received at McLean Hospital outside of Boston. During his time in treatment there, and while he was receiving insulin coma treatment, she also records that he was rational and coherent enough to be giving lectures on topics in mathematics and game theory to the medical staff and nurses, who obviously thought they were worth their time to attend.

Every medication given to him made him better, while he took them, which was basically only while he was in a hospital. He had multiple hospitalizations over many years but never took medication outside of a hospital. But only in the case of psychiatric illness could Nasar (or any other writer) get away with saying that his refusal to take antipsychotic medication "may have been fortuitous." She goes on to say that "such drugs, in a high percentage of cases, produce horrible, persistent symptoms like tardive dyskinesia-stiffening of head and neck muscles and involuntary movements, including of the tongue-and a mental fog, all of which would have made his gentle reentry into the world of mathematics a near impossibility"—as if he had been in something other than a "mental fog" for thirty years.

Antipsychiatry publications have seized on this speculative assertion made entirely without reference to a single study as evidence of the inevitable damaging effects of psychotropic medications—in other words, a political statement as opposed to a scientific one.

This is an interesting speculation and needs to be looked at more carefully. Nash believed that he "cured" himself using the methods of science and logic (i.e., mathematics). He was completely incapacitated for almost thirty years, but he felt he was eventually able to reject his "irrational hypotheses of delusional thinking" (p. 354). Reaching a stage in his illness where he accepts the premise that there's a condition to cure is certainly an advance. Why it took thirty years to accomplish this is anyone's guess, but, the risk of a debilitating tardive dyskinesia notwithstanding, would it not have been better for Nash and his family if he could have done something more than just be delusional and hallucinating for thirty years?

Nasar's position is common among those who don't have any responsibility for treating patients with schizophrenia or other serious mental illnesses. She makes the assumption that medications that actually helped him would somehow have been ultimately harmful and that not taking them conferred a kind of preservative function in his brain, which was later manifest as remission. The problem is that she offers absolutely no evidence in support of that assertion. There has never been a study that I'm aware of that remotely suggests that patients who don't take medication have better outcomes or are more likely to enter remission than those who do. There is plenty of evidence to the contrary. Only for psychiatric illnesses do we hypothesize that stopping the brain from behaving abnormally for thirty years is actually bad and allowing it to run amok somehow good. This thinking is consistent with the dominant belief in academic psychiatry in the middle part of the twentieth century, which was that psychiatric illness had nothing to do with the brain and is actually a manifestation of the soul (if it's not the brain, then what else are we talking about?).

If a patient had grand or petit mal seizures for thirty years, we would assume that trying to control them would be better than not. In conditions like diabetes, or even acne, we assume that treating is better for long-term health than not treating. Why isn't this the case for hallucinations, delusional beliefs, bizarre perceptual experiences, and cognitive distortions? These are NOT harmful to the brain? They are NOT indicative of abnormal neurochemical or neurophysiologic functioning? If a surgical patient ends up dead or severely debilitated after a "routine" surgery, why is that not as bad as a psychiatric patient with tardive dyskinesia, 99 percent of which are so mild such that the patient is usually unaware of having the problem, even when it's frequently pointed out to him or her (the condition is more common in women)?

Nasar is very impressed by Nash's remission. Had there been no remission, there would, of course, have been no book. Given his illness, the fact that he was able to go to Stockholm and receive the prize was a great triumph tastefully recorded in book and movie. The book goes into more detail about the Nobel committee's reservations about having Nash appear in Stockholm and giving him a microphone, not knowing what might come out of his mouth.

The "Beautiful Mind" in the title refers to the beauty of his extraordinary mathematical mind as it eventually emerged from the (certainly not drug-induced) mental fog of psychosis. But, while in remission, was Nash his old productive self? Was he "normal"? Could he work? Commenting on his recovery to an audience of psychiatrists in Madrid in 1996 regarding the "greatness" of his recovery, Nash said, "But maybe it is not such a great thing. Suppose you have an artist. He's rational. But suppose he cannot paint. He can function normally. Is it really a cure? Is it really a salvation? I feel I am not a good example of a person who recovered unless I can do some good work." He went on to add, mostly to himself, "Although I am rather old." Even if "recovered," Nash was no longer capable of productive work. From the age of thirty and older, he was completely dependent on others. The older textbooks in psychiatry, contrary to Nasar's implication, often referred to recovery. But many of these were labeled "recovery with defect." Although much improved, they were not back to their premorbid baseline and never would be. But Nasar is an economics correspondent for the New York Times and is not normally a medical writer.

On the other hand, neurologist Oliver Sacks, in his 1995 book An Anthropologist on Mars, in a chapter on frontal lobe dysfunction (The Last Hippie), continues the diatribe against psychotropic drugs in at least schizophrenia, likely a frontal or prefrontal lobe condition. While he was talking primarily about the patients he examined at a state psychiatric hospital who'd been lobotomized prior to the use of psychotropic drugs, he went on to say,

> Whether there is that much difference, neurologically or ethically, between psychosurgery and tranquillizers, is an uncomfortable question that has never really been faced. Certainly the tranquillizers, if given in massive doses may, like surgery, induce tranquility, may still the hallucinations and delusions of the psychotic, but the stillness they induce may be like the stillness of death-and, by a cruel paradox,

deprive the patients of the natural resolution that may sometimes occur with psychoses and instead immure in them a lifelong drug-induced illness.

The problem is, as usual, the treatment, not the illness. Sacks does not describe for us what these patients are like without this "induced tranquility," and he doesn't tell us how he manages schizophrenia in his patients over the course of twenty or thirty years, if he ever does.

While one can envy the poetic talents of an Oliver Sacks and his stature in the world of neurology for the masses, his emphasis and use of medical facts in the field of psychiatry suffer from the hubris of someone who feels that his knowledge in one field necessarily gives him expertise in every other. This is somewhat surprising in a book published as recently as 1995. Truth be told, his assertion that the ethics of tranquillizer use in psychiatry has never "really been faced" is incredible and, dare I say, irresponsible.

From residency training programs since my own in the later 1960s, when use of "powerful" medications for "mythical" conditions was questioned time and again, to numerous professional meetings and research studies over the past five decades, the issue has been very much addressed. Use of these medications is as ethical as any in any branch of medicine, because most patients benefit, often very substantially, and being mentally ill is not a condition as trivial as dandruff (dandruff sufferers may disagree). Certainly there are many patients who benefit very little from these medications, as in the treatment of many cancers, lupus, MS, ulcerative colitis, and countless degenerative diseases, but it is certainly not unethical to make some attempt to help. This is because so many do benefit from medication, especially when paired with other forms of treatment, such as psychotherapy and psychosocial rehabilitation.

Talking about medications in psychiatry is like the story of the blind men trying to describe an elephant. Since the conditions being treated are so varied, judgments about effectiveness depend on the medication, symptoms, and population. If one looks at cancer, for example, one diagnosis with one prognosis does not suffice for the entire spectrum of cancers and patients. Comparing survival rates for pancreatic and bronchogenic (lung) carcinomas will yield different results than what one might expect in basal cell (skin) cancers or early-stage colon cancers. Mental conditions, especially psychoses, vary in many of the same ways.

Dr. Sacks says he examined patients at a New York state psychiatric hospital in the 1970s and 1980s. The population he may have seen included those patients who were still left in the state hospitals after the advent of antipsychotic medication and still couldn't make it in the community. Maybe they were the chronic and persistently ill for whom medications were minimally effective and required "massive doses" (his words) to "induce tranquility" (his words again). Maybe it would have been better to just allow them to be and do whatever they were doing when not tranquillized. But to say that medication deprived them of "the natural resolution that may sometimes occur with psychoses and instead immure them in a lifelong drug-induced illness" makes good poetry but makes the unwarranted assumption that, before antipsychotic medications, there were somehow more spontaneous remissions than after these drugs were introduced. There is absolutely no evidence for that assertion.

The truth is that there are many, probably the great majority of patients, with the various forms of psychoses (schizophrenias, bipolars, and all varieties in between) whose lives are going to be considerably better and more rewarding and productive with medications than without.

Of course, it might be interesting to approach it from the Dr. Sacks perspective: *"Well, Mr. Doe, it's like this: In twenty-five or thirty years from now you have a 25 percent chance of spontaneous remission (of course, a 75 percent chance against) after which you might even be able to hold a job, well, probably not, but maybe. While we're waiting, plan on (in a relatively good scenario) ten or fifteen long hospitalizations in between which you may experience a few months of lucidity followed by periods of severe depression, with or without hallucinations. If you don't kill yourself intentionally in the first ten years of illness, maybe someone will kill you on the street, which is where you may end up after your friends, employers, and maybe even family have given up after one too many paranoid threats and one too many trashings of the house in one of your psychotic rages. Your younger siblings will move out as teenagers, because they resent your verbal and physical attacks on their person and their friends.*

"In a somewhat less optimistic scenario, maybe you spend twenty-five continuous years in a state psychiatric hospital, but only if you agree to stay, since you can sign out the minute you aren't homicidal or suicidal, no matter how

depressed or psychotic you are. Actually, forget that last scenario. In 1955, with at least a third less population, we had 560,000 state psychiatric beds but now only 40,000, so that's not an option today even if you wanted it.

"We do have what we call community integrated living arrangements (CILAs) now or nursing homes, both of which are (maybe) better than living in hospitals. They won't take you unless you can behave in a civil, nonviolent manner among other patients and staff. If you make a suicide attempt and fail to die, forget about the CILA or nursing home, since their legal council will advise them to not accept you because you're high risk. If you're not acceptable at home or in a boarding facility, the only option left is the Cook County Jail. Of course, you can't get in there by just being depressed or psychotic. You have to commit a crime. What? You were just protecting yourself from the KGB and CIA agents following you? Tell it to the judge, and see me again in twenty-five years if you get better and if you live that long.*

"Or we might try medication. Medication may allow you to stay in school or hold a job, live at home, or even support yourself or a family if you have one. However, some think that might be unethical, because, after all, there are certain risks (only drugs in psychiatry pose risks, of course) associated with their use. The trivial nature of your psychiatric condition makes the risk not worth taking. However, should you have something serious, like acne, then of course 'powerful drugs' (like Accutane) are worth the risk. After all, acne has lesions and is there for all the world to see, will make you feel bad about yourself, and we wouldn't like that, because feeling bad about yourself might make you sad."*

Exaggeration? Maybe a little. But if we look at the metaphorical elephant in its entirety, one is, in fact, likely to see many patients who do very well without "massive doses" of medication, who do not spend years in hospitals, and who, despite serious disorders, lead rather productive lives. Over the past forty-five-plus years, I've seen multiple examples of very ill teens and young adults who do considerably worse over time by not taking medications than by taking them. Most patients seen in adolescence or young adulthood have done very well over time and, with or without my approval and supervision, have tapered off medication. Some have done well, and some consistently decompensate. But of those who decompensate (like John Nash), many by this time with careers and mortgages and children to support, most choose to stay on. Based on the population of patients seen at Alexian Brothers during my tenure (certainly a better cross section of the psychiatrically ill population than Dr. Sachs's state hospital group), I've seen far more tragedies in those patients who've refused medications over the expanse of their illness than those who've taken them.

Today there are medications that make tardive dyskinesia, especially the much less common disabling form that in the general practice of psychiatry is rare, much less of a risk, and 99 percent of cases are so mild that the individuals deny having it at all, even with a formal diagnosis. Nevertheless, the issue today is the same that confronted John Nash in the 1950s and 1960s: Are the delusions, hallucinations, or disordered thinking signs of illness, or are they reality? No matter how good the medications or how free of side effects they become, many patients are simply not going to take them, convinced that what they're experiencing is truth and what others tell them is a lie.

Luckily, most psychiatric patients don't suffer from schizophrenia. Mood disorders, anxiety, and substance use disorders are far more common by a substantial degree. Are powerful drugs useful here? For these disorders, behavioral and psychotherapeutic techniques work best for the largest number, but for the most severe patients, "powerful drugs" can be, well, powerful, and that can be lifesaving.

Suicide

When psychiatric patients die, it's often by their own hands. Death by suicide generates different reactions in people depending on their relation to the deceased. To most people (who don't want to die), killing oneself seems inexplicable, tragic, and sometimes even immoral. In most disease states, the patient doesn't want to die and goes to a physician or surgeon for advice in preventing death (Dr. Kevorkian is an example of an exception that actually seems to prove the rule).

Suicide strikes many of us as either foreseeable (hence, seemingly preventable) or, more commonly, someone's "fault," depending on the circumstances. At some point after a successful suicide, an assignment of "fault" will be made. A mother whose son commits suicide may blame her daughter-in-law if there were marital problems. The person who committed suicide may leave a note absolving his parents, wife, or friends of any fault in his death, thereby leaving them to wonder if this was his way of actually blaming them. Parents or children will invariably blame themselves for not seeing it coming or not finding a way to prevent it, all the more so if the suicide comes in the context of the sudden loss of a child, spouse, or job. In most plays, movies, or novels, a suicide is always seen as a more or less inevitable outcome of the main character's "failure" to deal with his challenges, especially when created by himself. In Greek tragedy, the problem is the main character's (usually a kind of everyman) tragic inability to escape the clutches of "fate," no matter how gallant the struggle (e.g., Oedipus Rex).

But in the real world, most completed suicides are the result of mental illness. These are usually seen without the literary or artistic imagery and without any comprehensible cause other than the illness itself, sometimes associated with varying degrees of social, interpersonal, or professional "failure." If the person was in some form of therapy, then those left behind may see the doctor or therapist to be "at fault," since, in the view of some family members, suicide is a preventable occurrence, and the sole purpose of treatment, in their eyes (not necessarily the patient's), is to prevent death. This is especially so if the patient was admitted to a hospital specifically because of suicidal threats or, very often, some kind of suicide attempt. Once having threatened or attempted suicide, unless the disorder is successfully treated or the patient "cured," the disorder remains potentially lethal indefinitely. Therefore, it's in the acute psychiatric hospital environment that one sees those patients with the very highest mortality rates, much higher than at state hospitals, whose patients are generally more chronic. It is to the more local community psychiatric hospitals, like Alexian Brothers Behavioral Health with over six thousand high-risk admissions yearly, that patients come in voluntarily (or involuntarily) for treatment.

However, the patient may have a different view of what treatment means. From a rational (most admitted patients are not psychotic) patient perspective, treatment is seen as a process by which relief from suffering is attained. If the process fails, death may seem like peace and relief from torment. Most seriously depressed patients do not commit suicide, because they understand that those close to them may suffer. But one symptom of depression is the mind's distortion of thought such that the sufferers come to believe that their death will actually relieve the suffering of those who love them. If not working, patients will usually feel that they are sucking up the meager (the sufferer invariably sees poverty and destitution looming even in wealthy families) resources of the family, and death means more for the survivors, as if they were all floating on a lifeboat at sea. Suicide here seems a grand and noble act of familial love.

If the patient is so depressed that psychosis becomes part of the clinical picture, death may take on a religious or spiritual significance and be quite compelling. Hospitals, therapists, and medications may all be seen as malevolent attempts to prolong suffering and thwart the will of God toward this "sinner," though to say such things would result in more treatment and more interference with the will of God. The consequence of unsuccessful treatment is, as in lung cancer and cerebro-basilar degeneration (mentioned earlier) and countless other diseases, death.

While psychiatric illnesses seem so different from other lethal medical conditions, are they really? The good news is that the greatest majority of all psychiatric disorders are successfully treatable given time and resources. Even those who are not successfully treated are, for various reasons, unable to commit suicide, although they may never stop thinking about it. The bad news is a minority of patients who aren't treated successfully will choose to die; the majority of these are males who are less likely to seek or stay in treatment if unsuccessful.

No matter how many studies are published showing the inability of professionals to accurately predict suicide in individual cases (given the variability in patients and circumstances), the belief exists that suicide is, once treated by a professional, predictable and preventable. Don't think so?

Fifteen or twenty years ago, I attended an educational program sponsored by the Illinois Psychiatric Society on malpractice in psychiatry. One of the speakers that day was a rather well-known Chicago plaintiff's lawyer. His presentation was short and to the point. It went something like this: *If your patient commits suicide, no matter what the circumstances, then you'll very likely be sued.* End of story (it was not a long presentation). I wondered if he gave the same speeches to all the medical specialists. Did he give neurologists, oncologists, surgeons, and cardiologists the same spiel? After the program I asked him just that. As I suspected, he didn't say that in the same way to other specialists, because (although he's sued plenty of them), as he explained it, they have patients who have certain diseases that, even if treated, are expected to kill them, so bringing suit requires evidence of negligence in the treatment. In psychiatry, he explained, the patients are otherwise healthy and not expected to die, presumably having a condition that, in and of itself (e.g., being depressed or being psychotic) is not lethal. Of course, while a knowledgeable and able litigator, he is actually quite wrong. The error is in the apparent logic of the patient being "healthy." The patient is usually quite the opposite of healthy. Mentally "sick" can be quite the equal of or even far worse than physically sick (e.g., when others die along with the patient). Recall the earlier discussion of ECT regarding my father seen in the hospital by neighborhood friend Dr. James Jordan, who described him as looking, well, "sick." Was he "sick," or was it "psychological"? Even the distinction is, given rapidly expanding knowledge in neuroscience, artificial. It is a matter of fact that some of these patients will continue to die regardless of how conscientious or expert the care is, just as in the other specialties, because the illnesses being treated are just as real and, in certain cases, every bit as lethal.

Patients and families actually know this, which is why in most suicides (or attempted suicides where patients survive) where doctors know their patients and families even a little, lawsuits are not very common. A lawyer sees a skewed sample, and his job is to find a way to sue someone, even if a reason is not immediately apparent.

The goals of lawsuits in psychiatry are not different than in other specialties, though less common. The plaintiff's lawyer has to demonstrate a duty and then a dereliction of that duty owed to the patient, usually argued as a deviation from some presumed community standard of care. The "standard of care" is defined as what other doctors in the specialty being examined— in this case, psychiatry—would likely do in the case in question. Suits are probably more common among that smaller percentage of psychiatrists who work in a high-risk environment like a hospital, since that's where all the failed suicides and seriously depressed or psychotic patients end up, some of whom will have long and difficult treatment experiences.

Working in a hospital setting, we have seen that some psychiatrists who only see outpatients will refuse to continue to see patients who have attempted suicide. The reason here is the worry that they put themselves at greater risk of lawsuits by seeing high-risk patients. While this is true for all physicians who see very ill patients and is an accepted risk all physicians go to bed with daily, psychiatry is burdened with the unfortunate notion that mental illnesses occur in "healthy" patients who dwell under the not-expected-to-die illusion. But it is an illusion, since our patients—including those who refuse or do not fully cooperate with treatment, give it their all, and still fail to respond—experience incredible mental pain and suffering, and a certain number will choose to die rather than go on no matter what. So far, since suicide is often an impulsive act, no one has developed a valid, truly predictive formula.

In any lawsuit, the plaintiff's lawyer cannot assert the negligence claim. Someone with presumed similar expertise, like another psychiatrist (or surgeon or cardiologist), has to attest to the "negligence" or cite in what way the defendant physician has deviated from the "standard of care." If the case involves a neurosurgeon or an interventional cardiologist, the plaintiff's expert is supposed to have the same credentials and do the same procedures. In psychiatry, always the exception, the standards are not that strict. So while a defendant psychiatrist may work in a hospital and admit three hundred or more patients yearly and see suicidal patients on a daily basis, the plaintiff's "expert" may be a forensic specialist who spends most of his or her time examining patients awaiting trial or nonsuicidal patients in a part-time office. They may even admit one or two patients somewhere each year. In these cases we see the articulation of standards of care by those who have limited experience with the long-term management of treatment-resistant depression or psychosis. But despite the implication that suicide is prima facie evidence of negligence, in my limited experience as expert witness in cases like these, juries generally do not agree and usually find for the doctor.

The only way to guarantee that someone who does not respond to treatment remains alive is to guard that person in some closed environment indefinitely, a form of psychiatric life support. As mentioned in chapter 13, two or three days without verbalized suicidal intent is the latest criterion for denial, the treating doctor's opinion actually meaning very little. Managed care organizations deny based on their criteria, always pointing out that they don't make clinical decisions (depending on what the meaning of "is" is). State hospitals are vanishing, and even if they were still available or if managed care were less intrusive, until we find better ways of treating the treatment-resistant, suicides will continue to occur with greater frequency than we'd like and in surprisingly unpredictable fashion.

In 2002, I served on a committee of the American Psychiatric Association (APA), which was charged with the task of recommending whether or not the APA should develop guidelines for suicide assessment. Members of that committee were given a number of references to read, one of which was a report called "Safer Services," prepared by the British National Health Service. It was published in 1999 and was an in-depth review of all suicides and homicides and known suicide and homicide attempts by mentally ill persons occurring in Great Britain during the previous year. There were about five thousand deaths reviewed. The method was the "psychological post mortem." The conclusion of the report was that they could come to no firm conclusions, since it was not possible to reliably distinguish among those who ultimately went on to completed suicide from those who showed suicidal thoughts but did not make attempts. The APA did go on to recommend guidelines, however, since members preferred weak guidelines to none at all.

Homicide

Another trouble with psychiatry is dealing with the unpredictability of a patient's social behavior. For example, when a psychiatric patient makes the national news, it's seldom for something good. At times like these there are always attempts to assign blame, and sometimes it's a psychiatrist (or psychiatry as a profession) to blame for failing to predict the likelihood of a particular act in a specific person. The fact that there are no data supporting the claim that we can make such predictions is apparently no deterrent. A case in point is that of one John Hinckley, who in 1982 shot President Ronald Reagan outside a hotel in Washington, DC. Hinckley had a fantasied relationship with movie star Jodi Foster, who, at the time, was a student at Yale. His goal was to somehow get her attention and admiration by doing something dramatic. As we all know, he succeeded.

He had apparently been seeing a psychiatrist in his hometown in Colorado for some time prior to going to Washington, DC, to shoot the president. Of course, he didn't tell his doctor that he was planning to do something like this, but that didn't prevent his doctor from being sued for "negligence" by one of the injured parties. The suit never went anywhere, since it was going to be extremely difficult to argue that, among the tens of thousands of patients (and nonpatients) who have fantasied relationships with movie stars and other celebrities, Hinckley's psychiatrist somehow could have or should have been able to predict that behavior in his patient and either "cure" (a truly silly word in most of medicine) him or, at the least, warn the authorities and potential victims.

I bring up this example, because as luck would have it, a few days after the shooting I was bringing my twelve-year-old son to a visit with his orthopedic surgeon. He suffered from a deficiency of oxygen to his brain when his end of the placenta that he and his twin brother were attached to separated prematurely (placenta previa) from his mother's uterus while being born. The result is a condition referred to generically as cerebral palsy. "Palsy" is an old-fashioned word for paralysis. Damage to the motor areas of the brain is reflected in paralysis or at least varying degrees of motor dysfunction in the body. In my son's case, the problem presented primarily as spasticity and weakness in his legs and weakness in his arms.

In the absence of proper electrical influence from the brain to the muscles of the body, life with cerebral palsy is a lifelong struggle to prevent the progressive advancement of motor spasticity. Orthopedic surgeons step in as the patient progressively loses the battle to prevent advancing spasticity by cutting some of the spastic muscles, allowing them to "lengthen," so some walking, however unsteady, can become possible. His first hamstring "lengthening" surgery was at age five (his heel cords were done earlier), and he started walking at that time. He went on to have a few more surgical procedures over several years.

During the visit his surgeon, commenting on the Hinckley case, casually volunteered, "You know, nowadays we (orthopedic surgeons) like to talk about curing people." His point (paraphrased) was: "When are you psychiatrists going to be able to fix people like we do?" My reply was "I am overjoyed that you have a plan to cure my son. I was not expecting a cure, but if you can we'll certainly welcome it." His facial expression changed from slightly superior to slightly embarrassed, and he obviously got the point. He was (and may still be) a very good surgeon who obviously wasn't going to cure anyone with cerebral palsy, but what he did do over the preceding seven years (and later) was greatly appreciated. If we'd come to see him expecting "cure," we'd be setting up ourselves (and him) for ultimate disappointment.

Orthopedic surgeons "cure" broken bones, and they "treat," with varying degrees of success, other conditions. They're great to have available when you need them.

The more recent mass shootings at Sandy Hook School and in a Colorado theater raise questions again about mental illness and what can be accomplished with mentally ill patients. These discussions are merely a futile form of public hand wringing focused basically on how to prevent mentally ill people from killing us normals.

As a psychiatrist, I know that the only reliable predictions I can make about anyone's future behavior is to look at past behavior. In the two incidents cited above, neither person had killed previously, nor does any amount of exposure to violent video games (the National Rifle Association blamed violent video games, but they're just as popular in Japan, England, and France, but the actual killing is more common here) or lust for macabre movies predict these behaviors. There are millions who do the same and never hurt anyone.

As a society we're not about to go back to a psychiatry-as-Big-Brother-surrogate persona that, if it ever did exist, is not about to reappear. Psychiatry is not going to be able to prevent the mass killings we've seen at Sandy Hook and in Colorado, because we don't know how to, and those who could do the job (Congress, gun control) choose not to, so we look foolish acting like we know when we don't.

Neuroplasticity

The Cartesian dualism in psychiatry over the years has been based on a fundamental error. It was as if "biological" or "genetic" meant hardwired and invariable when it came to human emotional life, and "learned" implied something in the brain that was created but not present to start with. This, it turned out, was an incredibly naive way of looking at human biology, but it explains why the psychiatry residents at Harvard when Dr. Kandel was there found it so difficult to find a psychiatrist in Boston who knew anything (or cared) about genetics. The variability in humans, individually and culturally, speaks loudly to the fact the learning plays a major role in the development of humans. All of this leads us back to Kandel's five principles mentioned in chapter 10, which bear repeating:

1. All mental processes are neural.
2. Genes and their protein products determine neural connections.
3. Experience alters gene expression.
4. Learning changes neural connections
5. Psychotherapy (and education/learning) changes gene expression.

As a child/adolescent psychiatry resident at UCLA in 1968, I had the opportunity to learn about research being done at the UCLA Brain Research Institute (BRI). I was fortunate to have one lecture given to me by Dr. Arnold Scheibel. Dr. Scheibel continues to be honored by an annual Arnold Scheibel Lecture and Prize at UCLA, given each year by a graduate student in neuroscience.

Dr. Scheibel began his medical career with an initial interest in cardiology but was impressed by the pervasiveness of emotional factors in cardiovascular illness. That led him to switch to psychiatry. However, he was concerned about the lack of knowledge about brain substrates in psychiatric illnesses in those years (early 1950s). He eventually studied neurophysiology at the Illinois Neuropsychiatric Institute prior to taking a position at UCLA in the departments of psychiatry and anatomy in 1955. By the time I arrived in 1968, he had become one of a very few psychiatrists/neuroscientists in the country, although UCLA actually had several.

It was at this lecture that I first learned about the concept of neuroplasticity, which is now one of the hottest areas of interest and research in psychiatry, neurology, and psychology. Scheibel studied brain microstructure. What he was able to demonstrate were changes in the structure of neurons in the brain of genetically similar mice by changing only the environment and experiences of experimental subjects and controls. Experimental animals were raised in "enriched" environments wherein they were given mazes and other "educational" tasks to learn and were then handled more by the research staff. Both groups were given the same diets, and both had opportunities to live together in social groups and allowed to do whatever "normal" mice like to do. After a time (I can't recall how long), their brains were examined, and there were (under the microscope) measurable structural differences. This was a time before PET scans and other neuroimaging techniques.

On microscopic examination it was dramatically evident that the dendrites (the part of the neuron that receives stimulation from other neurons before sending it through the cell body and down the axon to other neurons) of experimental animals were much more numerous and more robust than in the control animals. The dendrites of experimental animals showed more connections between the neuron (nerve cell) and other neurons in the neighborhood. The "education" these mice were getting was having some influence on the actual cellular structure of brain cells. "Experience" and/or "education" appeared to be having demonstrable influence on the very structure (and function?) of brain cells.

Today we would say that there is, in fact, a dynamic interplay between environment and how a given gene expresses itself. Scheibel's experiments antedated imaging studies that now can show the influence of experience in the brain in real time in living subjects. Today it is much more obvious that the brain is constantly changing or "remodeling" itself based on how experience influences gene expression and hence its actual physical structure. Genetics is not necessarily destiny, but neither can it be ignored. It has also become more evident that psychiatric conditions have negative influences on the brain in real time (Bourne). We have no choice but to try to do something about that once we find out more precisely how it all works. Kandel's Nobel Prize represents and validates the work of neuroscientists like Scheibel by showing that the mysterious workings of the mind, like memory, are associated with structural change (Kandel 2006). Soon other mysterious workings of the mind, like depression and psychosis, will be shown to be associated with structural and functional changes (i.e., the "lesions" that Thomas Szasz claimed weren't there).

EPILOGUE

So how does a hospital go from obscurity to the seventh largest (psychiatric) corporate entity in the country? Perhaps it wasn't so much that we were successful as much as the fact that others were unsuccessful or didn't see any point in staying with this bizarre calling. Certainly the national hospital companies that appeared in the 1960s and went out of business in the 1990s felt that the profit margins in psychiatry were no longer attractive, cut their losses, and went on to other things. Managed care turned out to be successful in destroying those programs whose financial viability rested firmly on a long-term treatment model that no one could afford to pay for anymore. Managed care didn't stop there and continues to be successful at wearing down the willingness of even nonprofit organizations to continue to treat psychiatric patients. For many it just isn't worth the trouble.

When a managed care company calls and demands that a doctor increases or changes a medication, one realizes that one is not the doctor in this situation but merely the vassal of an insurance company: "Call by 2:00 p.m., or we deny …" "Stop doing whatever you're doing (like seeing patients), and call by eleven or we deny." And on it goes. "So the patient was suicidal at 10:00 a.m. today, but was he suicidal at 4:00 p.m.? He was threatening to kill his mother on the phone today, and he tried to kill her before admission when she called the police, but can you say he'll really kill her if he went home tonight?" "Doctor, we're going to deny the first three days in the hospital, because he received no medication. He refused? You don't use injectables at Alexian Brothers anymore. Hmmm …" What sane person wants to do this?

The problem is that the patients keep coming—all the more since there are now fewer options out there for them, public or private. Managed care has been so successful at squeezing psychiatric programs that patients are boarding, as we saw in chapter 1, in emergency rooms all over the country. In the Alexian system there are two general hospitals within ten miles of each other that have discovered that it's cheaper for them to pay the Alexian Brothers Behavioral Health Hospital to care for unfunded psychiatric patients clogging up their emergency rooms than to keep them waiting for state hospital psychiatric beds that never seem to be available. Patients like it better, as well. The problem is having a bed available for anyone regardless of payer, and that meant the added inconvenience (and expense) of sending eight-hundred-plus patients to other locations.

But good intentions and the loss of some competitors are probably not enough to explain how Alexian Brothers Behavioral Health got to number seven in the nation. The purchase of a hospital that was losing $250,000 a month in 1999 was a move that said something about the Alexian Brothers' willingness to commit resources to psychiatry. While Mark Frey was, in my opinion, the primary reason for our relatively favorable position in the 1990s, when HCA/Woodland was purchased in 1999, Mr. Frey was working as CEO at another psychiatric hospital for the previous eighteen months. The Alexian Brothers had committed to psychiatry, whether he was coming back or not. Getting him back, however, was a major factor in the hospital's subsequent growth. He was chiefly responsible for the financial viability of the psychiatry division from 1990 to 1997, and, despite all the challenges, he found a way to keep it profitable enough to give the Brothers a reason to spend $10 million to buy and remodel the hospital building that became Alexian Brothers Behavioral Health Hospital in 1999. Under Mark Frey the hospital became profitable enough to expand from 95 inpatient beds to 141 currently with eight separate inpatient units. Under him also, the day hospital programs expanded to eight discreet programs as it became evident that "one size fits all" was not going to suit the needs of those who came to us for help.

Stability of leadership over time may also have been a factor in convincing the Brothers and hospital administration to feel comfortable with their investment in psychiatry. They agreed to stay with the program during the many changes and challenges during the years when managed care devastated many programs in the area. Dr. Greg Teas joined the staff at Alexian Brothers in 1976, and I came there in 1977. Dr. Mike Rogers was instrumental in recruiting both of us and stayed around for several years as mentor after he resigned as chair. Mark Frey arrived at the same time to work in the adolescent program.

In the early 1980s, Francine McGouey was hired as a teacher on the adolescent unit, later to become chief operating officer (COO) when Mark Frey was rehired as CEO of the new psychiatric hospital in 1999. Like Mark Frey, Francine was not content to just do her job and leave. She started as a special education teacher in the adolescent program but somehow became interested in the quality improvement process as it applied to psychiatric hospitals. A very bright "systems" thinker from the start, she became a highly effective COO when the hospital opened under the Alexian Brothers logo in 1999. When Mark Frey was promoted to CEO of the entire Alexian Health System in 2007, Francine was promoted from COO to CEO a short time later. Under her leadership the hospital remained financially viable, and the hospital's programs continued to grow. When she retired in 2011, Clay Ciha became CEO. Mark Frey had recruited Clay into a marketing position in 1999, and he took over the health system's neuroscience division when Frey became CEO of the health system in 2007.

Dr. Greg Teas has been a major constant at the hospital since the 1970s and in 2011 took over as chief medical officer (CMO). A subspecialist in addictions, he headed the addictions treatment programs at the hospital for at least fifteen years, is a past president of the American Academy of Clinical Psychiatrists (an organization that originated at Washington University, St. Louis), and has been a powerful intellectual/scientific influence at the hospital for almost forty years. He's served on the Medical Relations Committee at Alexian Brothers Medical Center for years before and after Alexian Brothers Behavioral Health came into existence and is a pretty good golfer and first-rate human being (at least when he's not golfing).

Finally, I have always felt that another important factor in the hospital's growth and ability to compete has been the willingness of the Alexian administration to avoid the temptation, always present during times of stressful change, to micromanage the psychiatric division. There is nothing that stifles creativity and initiative more in good employees than trying to do their thinking for them. Before 1999, maybe it was because we were across a four-lane road from the Alexian Brothers Medical Center and somewhat isolated from the day-to-day general hospital goings-on. Maybe it was because we were psychiatry, and we're supposed to be inscrutable anyway. Whatever it was, we were given fairly free reign to do what we thought was in the best interest of our programs, and in the end, I think we were right. After 1999, with now a separate hospital of our own and a CEO (Mr. Frey) who didn't like being managed at all, growth continued. In 2014, with demand still high, twenty-four more beds were added in Elk Grove, and in 2015 to 2016 more expansion was on the drawing board in the form of residential programs for substance abuse and anxiety disorders in addition to the expansion of the psychiatric division occasioned by the Alexian partnership with the Adventist system known as Amita Health and a merger with another health system.

The future is a difficult thing to predict. Managed care, as practiced in psychiatry, currently simply cannot last. If it does, psychiatry's future doesn't look very good, since the psychiatric patient tends to draw the short straw. Even as we speak, the Trump administration is working hard to disrupt health benefits for the poor and seems to be succeeding. But hopefully the trend toward extinction has at least been attenuated.

REFERENCES

Abelson, J. L., Curtis, G. C., Sagher, O., Albucher, R. C., Harrigan, M., Taylor, S. F., Martis, B., Giordani, B. (2005). Deep brain stimulation for refractory obsessive-compulsive disorder. *Biological Psychiatry, 57*(5), 510-516. doi:10.1016/j.biopsych.2004.11.042

Abrams, R. (1997). *Electroconvulsive Therapy.* New York: Oxford University Press

Abrams, R., & Essman, W. (Eds) (1982). *Electroconvulsive Therapy: Biological foundations and clinical applications.* New Delhi: Spectrum Publishing

Arnedo, J., Svrakic, D. M., Del Val, C., Romero-Zaliz, R., Hernandez-Cuervo, H., Molecular Genetics of Schizophrenia, Consortium, Fanous, A. H., Pato, M. T., Pato, C. N., de Erausquin, G. A., Cloninger, C.R., Zwir, I. (2015). Uncovering the hidden risk architecture of the schizophrenias: confirmation in three independent genome-wide association studies. *American Journal of Psychiatry, 172*(2), 139-153. doi:10.1176/appi.ajp.2014.14040435

Ban, T. A. (2007). Fifty years chlorpromazine: a historical perspective. *Neuropsychiatric Disease and Treatment, 3*(4), 495

Bargmann, C.I. & Lieberman, J.A. (2014). What the brain initiative means for psychiatry. *American Journal of Psychiatry, 171*(10) 1038-1040.

Barahal, H. S. (1958). 1000 Prefrontal Lobotomies: A five to ten year follow-up. *Psychiatric Quarterly, 32*(4) 652-678.

Berlioz, Hector (1990) Medical Studies, Paris 1821. In *The Memoirs of Hector Berlioz*, 1803-1865, trans. and ed. David Cairns, London, England: Cardinal

Bettelheim, B. (1967). *The empty fortress: Infantile autism and the birth of the self*. New York, NY: Free Press

Bettelheim, B. (1956). Schizophrenia as a reaction to extreme situations. *American Journal of Orthopsychiatry*, 26(3) 507-518.

Bonner, T. N. (1991). *Medicine in Chicago, 1850-1950: A chapter in the social and scientific development of a city*. Chicago, Illinois: University of Illinois Press

Bourne, C., Aydemir, O., Balanza-Martinez, V., Bora, E., Brissos, S., Cavanagh, J. T,. et al. (2013). Neuropsychological testing of cognitive impairment in euthymic bipolar disorder: an individual patient data meta-analysis. *Acta Psychiatrica Scandinavica*, 128(3), 149-162. doi:10.1111/acps.12133

Burdett, H. C. (1891). *Hospitals and asylums of the world: Asylum construction, with plans and bibliography*. London, England: J & A Churchill

Chicago Medical Society (1922). *A History of medicine and surgery and physicians and surgeons of Chicago*. Chicago, Illinois. The Biographical Publishing Corporations

Clapesattle, E. (1941). *The doctors Mayo*. Minneapolis, Minnesota: Mayo Clinic

Coffey, C. E., Weiner, R. D., Djang, W. T., Figiel, G. S., Soady, S. A., Patterson, L. J., Holt, P. D., Spritzer, C. E., Wilkinson, W. E. (1991). Brain anatomic effects of electroconvulsive therapy. A prospective magnetic resonance imaging study. *Archives General Psychiatry*, 48(11), 1013-1021.

Collier, P. & Horowitz, D. (1984). *The Kennedys*. New York: Summit Books

Cosgrove, R. and Rausch, S., Website of THE FUNCTIONAL AND STEREOTACTIC NEUROSURGERY DIVISION, Massachusetts General Hospital and Harvard Medical School

Dahl, D. (2012) archivist, Alexian Brothers Archives. Illinois

D'Agostino, A. (1975). Depression: Schism in contemporary psychiatry. *American Journal of Psychiatry, 132*(6) 629

Davidson, L. (1990). *The Alexian Brothers of Chicago*. New York: Vantage Press

DeMyer, M. K., Barton, S., DeMyer, W. E., Norton, J. A., Allen, J., & Steele, R. (1973). Prognosis in autism: a follow-up study. *Journal of Autism and Child Schizophrenia, 3*(3), 199-246.

Deniker, P., Delay, J., Harl, J.M. (1952). Utilisation en therapeutique psychiatrique d'une phenothiazine d'action centrale elective. *Annals of Medicine and Psychology, 110*, 112-117.

Deniker, P. (1970) Introduction of neuroleptic chemotherapy into psychiatry. Ayd, F., Blackwell, B. (eds). *Discoveries in Biological Psychiatry*, 155-164, Baltimore: Ayd Medical Communication.

Diniz, B. S., Machado-Vieira, R., & Forlenza, O. V. (2013). Lithium and neuroprotection: translational evidence and implications for the treatment of neuropsychiatric disorders. *Neuropsychiatr Dis Treat, 9*, 493-500. doi:10.2147/NDT.S33086

Drasga, R.E. & Einhorn, L.H. (2014). Why oncologists should support single-payer national health insurance. *Journal of Oncology Practice, 10*(1), 7-11.

DuClaux, E. (1920). *Pasteur: The history of a mind* (English translation, 2013). London, England: W. B. Saunders Co

Dukart, J., Regen, F., Kherif, F., Colla, M., Bajbouj, M., Heuser, I., Frackowiak, R.S., Draganski, B. (2014). Electroconvulsive therapy-induced brain plasticity determines therapeutic outcome in mood disorders. *Proceedings of the National Academy of Sciences, 111*(3), 1156-1161. doi:10.1073/pnas.1321399111

Eisenberg, L. (1956). The autistic child in adolescence. *American Journal of Psychiatry, 112,* 607-612

Fink, M. (1979). *Convulsive therapy: theory and practice.* New York: Raven Press

Fink, M., Kety, S., McGaugh, J., Williams, T. (1974). *Psychobiology of convulsive therapy.* Washington D.C.: V.H. Winston & Sons

Flexner, A. (1910). *Medical Education in the United States and Canada.* New York: Carnegie Foundation Bulletin #4

Freeman, W., (1957). A follow-up study of 3000 patients. *American Journal of Psychiatry, 113,* 877-886.

Freud, S. (1974). *Cocaine Papers.* R. Byck, (Ed). New York: Stonehill Publishing Co.

Freud, S. (1974). *Cocaine Papers.* R. Byck, (Ed). London, England: Stonehill Publishing Co.

Freud, S., Breuer, J. (1895). *Studies in hysteria,* English translation by James Strachey printed 1957, New York: Basic Books

Freud, S. (1900). *The interpretation of dreams.* English translation by A.A.Brill, (1913). New York: The MacMillan Co.

Freud, S. (1961) *Civilization and its discontents.* James Strachey translation from the 1930 German publication. New York: Hogarth Press

Freud, S. (1961) *The future of an illusion.* James Strachey translation from the 1927 German publication. New York: Hogarth Press

Freud, S. (1961) *Moses and monotheism.* James Strachey translation from the 1939 German Publication. New York: Hogarth Press

Freud, S. (1917) Mourning and melancholia. In the *Collected Papers,* (4) p. 164, Joan Riviere translation, 1950. London, England: Hogarth Press

Freud, S. (2002). *The Schreber case.* Phillips, A (Ed). London, England: Penguin Books

Freud, S. (1968) *Infantile cerebral paralysis.* Lester Russin (trans). Coral Gables: Ineversity of Miami Press

Gildengers, A. (2013, August). The Neuroprotective Effects of Lithium. In S.A. Jacobson (Chair), *Advances in Geriatric Psychopharmacology.* Symposium conducted at the meeting of the American Psychiatric Association, San Francisco, CA.

Gorman, A. (2011, December 1) *Cedars-Sinai to cut most psychiatric services.* Los Angeles Times. Retrieved from http://articles.latimes.com/2011/dec/01/local/la-me-cedars-mental-20111201

Gortvay, G., Zoltan, I. (1966) *Semmelweis: His life and work.* Akademiai Kiadol, Budapest (English translation, 1968, as referenced in Encyclopedia Brittanica, 1980)

Greenberg, B. D., Gabriels, L. A., Malone, D. A., Jr., Rezai, A. R., Friehs, G. M., Okun, M. S., . . . Nuttin, B. J. (2010). Deep brain stimulation of the ventral internal capsule/ventral striatum for obsessive-compulsive disorder: worldwide experience. *Molecular Psychiatry, 15*(1), 64-79. doi:10.1038/mp.2008.55

Healy, D. (2004) *Explorations in a new world. The Creation of Psychopharmacology.* Boston, MA: Harvard Press.

Healy, D. (1998). Pioneers in Psychopharmacology. *International Journal of Neuropsychopharmacology, 1*(2), 191-194. doi:10.1017/S146114579800114X

Himmelstein, D. U., Jun, M., Busse, R., Chevreul, K., Geissler, A., Jeurissen, P., . . . Woolhandler, S. (2014). A comparison of hospital administrative costs in eight nations: US costs exceed all others by fa *Health Affairs, 33*(9), 1586-1594. doi:10.1377/hlthaff.2013.1327

Himmelstein, D., Woolhandler, S., Hellander, I. (2001) *Bleeding the Patient.* Philadelphia, PA: Common Courage Press

History of Health Insurance Benefits (2002, March). *Employee Benefit Research Institute.* Retrieved from: www.ebri.org

Huber, G., Gross, G., Schuttler, R., & Linz, M. (1980). Longitudinal studies of schizophrenic patients. *Schizophrenia Bulletin, 6*(4), 592-605.

International College of Surgeons, Surgical museum brochure, Chicago

Kalinowsky, L. (1984). Biologic psychiatric treatments preceding pharmacotherapy. In F.J. Ayd and B. Blackwell, B. (Eds.), *Discoveries in Biological Psychiatry*, pp.59-67. Lippincott: Philadelphia, PA.

Kalinowsky, L. (1982) The history of electroconvulsive therapy. *Electroconvulsive Therapy: Biological Foundations and Clinical Applications.* New York: SP Medical & Scientific Books.

Kandel, E. (1998). A New Intellectual Framework for Psychiatry. *American Journal of Psychiatry, 155*(4), 457-469

Ibid. pp. 505-524

Kandel, E. R. (2004). The molecular biology of memory storage: a dialog between genes and synapses. *Bioscience Reports, 24*(4-5), 475-522. doi:10.1007/s10540-005-2742-7

Ibid. pp. 373

Kandel, Eric (2006). *In Search of Memory: The Emergence of A New Science of Mind.* New York, NY: W.W.Norton & Co.

Kanner, L. (1968). Autistic disturbances of affective contact. *Acta Paedopsychiatric, 35*(4), 100-136.

Kaufmann, C. (1976). *Tamers of Death.* New York, NY: Seabury Press.

Kaufmann, C. (1978) *The Ministry of Healing.* New York, NY: Seabury Press.

Kessler, R. (1996). *The Sins of the Father: Joseph P Kennedy and the Dynasty He Founded.* New York, NY: Warner Books.

Kety, S. S., Rosenthal, D., Wender, P. H., & Schulsinger, F. (1971). Mental illness in the biological and adoptive families of adopted schizophrenics. *American Journal of Psychiatry, 128*(3), 302-306. doi:10.1176/ajp.128.3.302

Kondziolka, D., Flickinger, J. C., & Hudak, R. (2011). Results following gamma knife radiosurgical anterior capsulotomies for obsessive compulsive disorder. *Neurosurgery, 68*(1), 28-32. doi:10.1227/ NEU.0b013e3181fc5c8b

Kraepelin, E. (1913). *Mixed Conditions of Maniacal-Depressive Insanity.* In T. Johnstone (Ed.), Lectures on Clinical Psychiatry, pp. 68-76. New York, NY: William Wood & Company.

Kutscher, B. (2013, November 16). Bedding Not Boarding. *Modern Healthcare.* Retried from http://www.modernhealthcare.com/article/20131116/MAGAZINE/311169992

Leamer, L.(1994). *The Kennedy Women: The Saga of an American Family.* New York, NY: Villard Books.

LeBow, B.(2002). *Health Care Meltdown.* Boise, ID: JRI Press.

Lehmann, H. E., & Hanrahan, G. E. (1954). Chlorpromazine; new inhibiting agent for psychomotor excitement and manic states. *Archives of Neurology & Psychiatry, 71*(2), 227-237.

Little, N.F. (1972). Early Years of McLean Hospital. Boston, MA: Francis A. Countway of Medicine.

Lovaas, O. I., Schreibman, L., & Koegel, R. L. (1974). A behavior modification approach to the treatment of autistic children. *Journal of Autism and Childhood Schizophrenia*, 4(2), 111-129.

Lozano, A. M., Mayberg, H. S., Giacobbe, P., Hamani, C., Craddock, R. C., & Kennedy, S. H. (2008). Subcallosal cingulate gyrus deep brain stimulation for treatment-resistant depression. *Biological Psychiatry*, 64(6), 461-467. doi:10.1016/j.biopsych.2008.05.034

May, P.R.A. (1968). *Treatment of Schizophrenia: A Comparative Study Of Five Treatment Methods*. New York, NY: Science House.

Mayberg, H. S. (1997). Limbic-cortical dysregulation: a proposed model of depression. *Journal of Neuropsychiatry & Clinical Neurosciences*, 9(3), 471-481. doi:10.1176/jnp.9.3.471

Mayberg, H. S., Brannan, S. K., Tekell, J. L., Silva, J. A., Mahurin, R. K., McGinnis, S., & Jerabek,.P. A. (2000). Regional metabolic effects of fluoxetine in major depression: serial changes and relationship to clinical response. *Biological Psychiatry*, 48(8), 830-843.

Mayberg, H. S., Liotti, M., Brannan, S. K., McGinnis, S., Mahurin, R. K., Jerabek, P. A., Silva, J. A., Tekell, J. L., Martin, C. C., Lancaster, J. L. & Fox, P. T. (1999). Reciprocal limbic-cortical function and negative mood: converging PET findings in depression and normal sadness. *American Journal of Psychiatry*, 156(5), 675-682. doi:10.1176/ajp.156.5.675

Mayberg, H. S., Lozano, A. M., Voon, V., McNeely, H. E., Seminowicz, D., Hamani, C., Schwalb, J. M., & Kennedy, S. H. (2005). Deep brain stimulation for treatment-resistant depression. *Neuron*, 45(5), 651-660. doi:10.1016/j.neuron.2005.02.014

McCullough, D. (2011) *The Greater Journey-Americans In Paris*. New York, NY: Simon & Schuster.

McCullough, D. (1977) The Path Between the Seas. New York, NY: Simon & Schuster.

Menninger, K. (1963) The Vital Balance. New York, NY: Vantage Press.

Miller, A. (1967). The lobotomy patient—a decade later: a follow-up study of a research project started in 1948. *Canadian Medical Association Journal,* 96(15), 1095-1103.

Modern Healthcare, (2010, March). *Largest Mental Health Providers.*

Modern Healthcare, (2012, February). *Largest Mental Health Providers.*

Mukherjee, S. (2011) *Cancer: Emperor of All Maladies.* New York, NY: Simon & Schuster.

Nasar, S. (1998). *A Beautiful Mind.* New York, NY: Simon & Schuster.

Noren, G., Rasmussen, S.A., Greenberg, B.D., Friehs, G., Chougule, P.B., Zheng, Z., & Epstein, M.H. (2002). Gamma Capsulotomy for Obsessive Compulsive Disorder. *Journal of Neurosurgery.*

Nunes, P. V., Forlenza, O. V., & Gattaz, W. F. (2007). Lithium and risk for Alzheimer's disease in elderly patients with bipolar disorder. Br J Psychiatry, 190, 359-360. doi:10.1192/bjp.bp.106.029868

Osler, W. (1921). The Evolution of Modern Medicine. New Haven, CT: Yale University Press.

Pagnin, D., de Queiroz, V., Pini, S., & Cassano, G. B. (2004). Efficacy of ECT in depression: a meta-analytic review. *Journal of ECT,* 20(1), 13-20.

Pollak, R. (1997). *The Creation of Dr. B: A Biography Of Bruno Bettelheim.* New York, NY: Simon & Schuster.

Porter, Roy (1997). *The Greatest Benefit to Mankind.* New York, NY: W.W. Norton & Co. New York.

(2006) *Psychiatry: An industry of death.* Documentary released on DVD. California: Citizens Commission On Human Rights (Church Of Scientology)

Rauch, S. L., Dougherty, D. D., Malone, D., Rezai, A., Friehs, G., Fischman, A. J., . . . Greenberg, B. D. (2006). A functional neuroimaging investigation of deep brain stimulation in patients with obsessive-compulsive disorder. *Journal of Neurosurgery, 104*(4), 558-565. doi:10.3171/jns.2006.104.4.558

Rosenthal, D., Wender, P. H., Kety, S. S., Welner, J., & Schulsinger, F. (1971). The adopted-away offspring of schizophrenics. *American Journal of Psychiatry, 128*(3), 307-311. doi:10.1176/ajp.128.3.307

Rutter, M., Greenfeld, D., & Lockyer, L. (1967). A five to fifteen year follow-up study of infantile psychosis. II. *Social and behavioural outcome. British Journal of Psychiatry, 113*(504), 1183-1199.

Sachs, O. (1995). *An Anthropologist on Mars.* New York, NY: Alfred A Knopf.

Safer Services (1999). *National Confidential Inquiry Into Suicides And Homicides By Persons With Mental Illness.* British National Health Service

Scofea, L.A. (1994). *The Development And Growth Of Employer-Provided Health Insurance. Monthly Labor Review, 117*(3), 3-10.

Shearer, James (1976) Master's Thesis

Shorter, E. (1997). A History of Psychiatry. New York, NY: John Wiley.

Shobe, F. and Gilder, M. (1968). A six to eighteen year follow-up of 27 private patients operated on 1951 to 1959. *The Journal of American Medical Association.* 206 (2): 327-332.

Small, I., Small, J., & Milstein, V. (1986). *Electroconvulsive Therapy.* In A. Silvano (Ed.), American Handbook of Psychiatry (Vol. 8). New York, NY: Basic Books.

Spadoni, A. (2012) Report To The Illinois Hospital Association

Sulloway, F. (1979). *Freud: Biologist of the Mind*. New York, NY: Basic Books.

Szasz, T. (1961). *The Myth of Mental Illness: Foundations of a Theory of Personal Conduct*. New York, NY: Harper & Row.

Taub, A., Lopes, A. C., Fuentes, D., et al. (2009). Neuropsychological outcome of ventral capsular/ventral striatal gamma capsulotomy for refractory obsessive-compulsive disorder: a pilot study. *Journal of Neuropsychiatry and Clinical Neuroscience, 21*(4), 393-397. doi:10.1176/appi. neuropsych.21.4.393.

Tendolkar, I., van Beek, M., van Oostrom, I., Mulder, M., Janzing, J., Voshaar, R. O., & van Eijndhoven, P. (2013). Electroconvulsive therapy increases hippocampal and amygdala volume in therapy refractory depression: a longitudinal pilot study. *Psychiatry Research, 214*(3), 197-203. doi:10.1016/j.pscychresns.2013.09.004

The International Exhibition of Sherlock Holmes. Royal College of Surgeons, Edinburgh, England

The History of Health Insurance In the United States, (2007) Northern California Neurosurgery Medical Group, www.neurosurgical.com

Toland, B. (April 27, 2014). How did America end up with this health system? *Pittsburg Post-Gazette*

Tooth, G.C. and Newton, M.P. (1961). *Leucotomy in England and Wales 1942-1954*. Great Britain Ministry of Health Reports on Public Health and Medical Subjects No. 104 (London: Her Majesty's Stationery Office, 1961).

Blumberg, A. and Davidson, A. (2009, Oct 22). Accidents of History Created U.S. Health System. In C. Watson (Executive Producer), *All Things Considered*. Washington, DC: National Public Radio.

Wender, P. H., Rosenthal, D., Kety, S. S., Schulsinger, F., & Welner, J. (1974). Crossfostering. A research strategy for clarifying the role of genetic and experiential factors in the etiology of schizophrenia. *Archives of General Psychiatry, 30*(1), 121-128.

Jeon, W. J., Kim, S. H., Seo, M. S., Kim, Y., Kang, U. G., Juhnn, Y. S., & Kim, Y. S. (2008). Repeated electroconvulsive seizure induces c-Myc down-regulation and Bad inactivation in the rat frontal cortex. *Experimental & Molecular Medicine, 40*(4), 435-444. doi:10.3858/emm.2008.40.4.435

Woolhandler, S., & Himmelstein, D. U. (2014). Administrative work consumes one-sixth of U.S. physicians' working hours and lowers their career satisfaction. *International Journal of Health Services, 44*(4), 635-642.

Zilboorg, G. (1941). *A history of medical psychology*. New York, NY: W.W.Norton & Co.

Printed in the United States
By Bookmasters